INDIVIDUALISED INTEGRATION

Studies of Deaf and Partially-hearing Children and Students in Ordinary Schools and Colleges

D.M.C. Dale

HODDER AND STOUGHTON
LONDON SYDNEY AUCKLAND TORONTO

British Library Cataloguing in Publication Data

Dale, D.M.C.
Individualised integration.
1. Deaf——Education——England
I. Title
371.91'2'0942 HV2716

ISBN 0-340-34260-9

First published 1984

Set in 11/12pt Bembo (Monophoto).

Printed and bound in Great Britain for
Hodder and Stoughton Educational,
a division of Hodder and Stoughton Ltd,
Mill Road, Dunton Green, Sevenoaks, Kent,
by Butler and Tanner Ltd
Frome and London

Contents

Foreword

If the integration of hearing-impaired children into ordinary classes is an idea whose time has come, Dr Dale may justly claim a crucial part in the conversion of that idea to actuality. Almost thirty years ago, when he first visited the United Kingdom to undertake postgraduate studies with Professor Sir Alexander Ewing, he began to formulate proposals for bringing children with severe auditory disabilities into closer contact with ordinary school life. The values of such contact for the children's progress in communication and for their social development were without doubt uppermost in his mind. After his return to New Zealand he was able to put into practice those initial plans. In 1965 he came to work permanently in the United Kingdom and from that time he has presented his case forcefully and persistently. As this book shows, he found education authorities who were willing to cooperate in bringing children who had previously been educated in special schools into the mainstream. Since then he has seen the trends in special education following in the direction of his cherished aims. A reduction in the numbers of pupils with severe and profound deafness has meant that the expense of providing special education in separate schools has become proportionately greater, and this at a time when education budgets have come under increased restraint. More importantly, and doubtless of greater long term significance, the tenor of professional thinking about the education of disabled children has grown much more sympathetic to Dr Dale's views. In the United Kingdom the Warnock Report of 1978 and recent legislation are indicative of this change. It is a change generally welcomed by parents and, happily, parental opinion itself is gaining increasing weight. In other countries too, as Dr Dale describes, a climate distinctly favourable to integration is now developing.

An extremely able teacher of deaf children, whose insight into their educational needs derives from many years of experience in special and in ordinary schools, Dale does not underestimate the exacting requirements which are to be met if an integrated education is to be better for the child than special school provision. In this text he gives practical and detailed information which is not available elsewhere and which will be most welcome to those teachers, both from the services for hearing-impaired children and from the ordinary schools, who recognise that the future is going to bring more deaf children into the ordinary school system.

Wilmslow, Cheshire
July 1983

H.L. Owrid

Figures

Tables

Preface

This book is written to encourage parents, teachers and educational and medical administrators to consider much greater individualised integration of deaf and partially hearing students into ordinary schools and colleges. Experiments and practices are reported here which have involved either transferring deaf and partially hearing students from special schools and units and placing them individually in their own local schools or colleges, or keeping them in their local ordinary schools and colleges without ever sending them to special facilities. Generous individual support has been found to be of crucial importance in many cases. Where hearing losses are not so severe, intelligence is above average, or homes are particularly supporting educationally, considerably less special treatment is required. Overall, per capita costs of individually integrated programmes are shown to be lower than for segregated or semi-segregated provision, and children, parents and teachers have been very much happier.

As well as emphasising the positive aspects of individualised special education programmes, evidence is reported of common difficulties which have been encountered in implementing this type of integration scheme.

Although most of the work reported here describes integration programmes for children and young people with defective hearing, a large proportion of the material is also relevant to those who work with children who have other special needs. Severe deafness is recognised as one of the most serious educationally handicapping conditions in children. In consequence, strategies and techniques which have been shown to be effective with them are usually felt to be highly successful with children who have sustained other handicaps. For example, blind and partially sighted children, physically handicapped, delicate and maladjusted boys and girls and those who are slow learners can certainly respond to most of the individual and micro-teaching-unit sessions which are recommended throughout this book. Parental involvement, home visiting, administrative aspects at the local education authority level, specific uses of support teachers and welfare assistants in both classrooms and resource rooms, and audio-visual and other teaching aids have all been found to be of benefit to other children with special needs.

The studies reported have immediate relevance for education authorities and for countries which do not at present have special schools or classes established, or who have insufficient facilities. All educational and medical administrators are urged strongly to consider this individualised approach with handicapped children before contemplating expensive day and residential schemes in specialist institutions and units.

Accommodation for those children who, for one reason or another, are required to live away from home, is also briefly considered. Again, however, the 'cottage home' form of residential care, near to the students' own homes, is shown to be more likely to provide a near-normal environment than the large, segregated institutional facilities which have so frequently been used during the past 200 years.

Advantages to unhandicapped children involved in well-organised integration programmes can be educational as well as social. Many children have become effective teachers while helping others who are handicapped and, in so doing, come to understand the topic under study much more as well as the effect of a handicapping condition: 'I read and I learn; I teach and I understand.' It is not always a one-way teaching process, of course. Deaf children can often help normally hearing ones with mathematics or art, map work, technical drawing and so on, and sometimes younger or less gifted children with language subjects.

Enabling ordinary children to learn at first hand about others who are less fortunate than themselves is felt to help to develop a more caring and better adjusted community. Good integration programmes enable unhandicapped children to develop both respect and affection for others and generally to learn to tolerate variability in society.

The concept of educating handicapped children and young adults in their own local schools and colleges has always been a tantalising one to many parents, teachers and doctors. With ample specialist backing, with modern technology and teaching methods, and as knowledge and experience increase, the possibility of providing various forms of such individually integrated education for all but a handful of hearing-impaired children and students, and probably most of those with other handicaps, has become a very real one.

PART I

Introductory

1

Current trends and emphases

Education in ordinary schools and colleges

In France, the United States, Canada, India, Italy, Scandinavia and the United Kingdom, legislation has recently been passed which strongly recommends the education of handicapped children in ordinary school classes wherever possible.[84,88,89] In 1978, the Report of the Committee of Enquiry into the Education of Handicapped Children and Young People in the United Kingdom (Chair.: Mrs H.M. Warnock)[232] stated: 'This is the central contemporary issue in special education which has been debated far beyond the frontiers of the education service. Educating handicapped and non-handicapped children together is the expression of a widely held and still growing conviction, that as far as is humanly possible, handicapped people should share the opportunities for self-fulfilment enjoyed by other people.'

Section 10 of the United Kingdom Education Act of 1976 had stated that, at some point in the future, all, or nearly all, handicapped children should be educated in ordinary schools. The Warnock Report regarded this legislation as a challenge to the education system as a whole and urged that it be taken seriously by everyone associated with education.

Statements such as these three are illustrations of the growing interest of senior research psychologists and principals of deaf schools in the question of integrated education programmes. 'The modern trend for all the handicapped is to try to keep them in their own homes and districts rather than segregate them in institutions' (Townsend[225]). In 1968, Tizard[220] asked:

> Is it *ever* possible to give handicapped children who spend most of their young lives in special schools . . . the range of experience which will enable them to live satisfying lives in the ordinary world? Or, to put the question the other way: is it possible to provide in ordinary schools the specialised services that handicapped children require while at the same time ensuring that they mix socially and in school with the ordinary children from their neighbourhood?

By 1971, Connor[43] was predicting that '... one of the next large scale movements in the education of the deaf in this country [the United States] will be an increased emphasis placed on meaningful and effective regular school programmes for deaf children'.

A number of parents, teachers and research workers have for some time questioned whether the advantages for many children of teacher specialisation in segregated institutions are not outweighed by the abnormal social situation.[16,44,48,52,86] Head teachers of special schools, however, can usually cite a number of cases of children who have been placed in ordinary schools without adequate support and have later been brought to them after having failed. A Ministry of Education report in 1963[158] also rightly criticised the practice of transferring hearing-impaired children from special schools and units to ordinary schools where special educational assistance was not available. After cautioning against such placements, however, a DES report,[73] in its final paragraph, stated: 'As knowledge grows and services improve, so too will the opportunities for integrating handicapped children in ordinary schools. The process is likely to accelerate, and new experimental forms of organisation are currently being made ...'

An amendment in 1968 to the Vocational Education Act (USA) provided that 10 per cent of the money supplied by the US Government at the state and local levels should be used for educating handicapped people. As a result, many community colleges throughout the US felt able to initiate programmes for their deaf students rather than send them long distances to the large national centres. The development of main-streamed programmes since 1968, stimulated by the Public Law 94-142 which provided for equal opportunities for all handicapped people, has been very considerable.[37]

In England, prior to the 1976 Education Act, studies had shown that the prevalence of handicaps sufficiently severe to cause educational retardation in children was as high as one in five.[72,194] The Department of Education and Science had therefore stated that 'the major responsibility for providing special education for the large number of children whose disabilities are less severe falls quite properly on ordinary primary and secondary schools'.[73] It went on (page 3): 'But opinion today is coming increasingly to favour the integration into ordinary schools of more of the severely handicapped children who are usually placed in special schools.' In round figures, the number of children issued with hearing aids were placed as follows: attending ordinary schools individually in the United Kingdom in December 1975, 10,500 (56%); attending units in ordinary schools, 1500 (8%); and attending day and residential schools for deaf and partially hearing children 6700 (36%).[77] Peripatetic (advisory) teachers of the deaf, by assisting parents of pre-schoolers and teachers in ordinary schools, have undoubtedly contributed to building up the number of individually integrated children.[52,75]

Since the late 1960s, an increasing number of workers have actively sought ways of meeting each handicapped person's special educational and social needs while *minimally* disrupting his or her everyday life. It is generally felt that, since the majority of these children will live and work in society, there is a need for them, during childhood, to have first-hand experience of ordinary society and for ordinary society to have first-hand experience of them. This has proved difficult when groups of deaf children attend ordinary schools.[56]

Some significant current practices

At the Lexington School in New York City, which has 350 deaf children enrolled, various types of integration programmes have been developed since 1968. By 1975, over 100 severely deaf children had transferred full-time from this school into ordinary school programmes by the age of 15, and were being offered follow-up assistance by itinerant teachers of the deaf; 50 per cent of all deaf infants had entered ordinary nursery schools and 40 per cent of all the children were going out to ordinary schools by the age of 12.[44]

In New Zealand in 1973, 110 children were transferred from schools and units for deaf and partially hearing children to their local ordinary schools (*see* chapter 6). Ages ranged from 6.5 to 16.9 years and hearing losses from 40 to 100 decibels (dB). Eight itinerant teachers of the deaf visited these children once, twice or three times each week for up to a quarter of each school day. In six of the 58 cases seen by the writer in 1976, much more specialist assistance was recommended, and in other cases, at least one more weekly visit was felt to be necessary. It was interesting, however, that only one child indicated that she was somewhat happier in her previous school, and none was recommended to return.

In Britain, of 301 children fitted with hearing aids in Norfolk in April 1977, fewer than 20 per cent had been sent to units or residential schools for deaf children.[52] Support was given to 239 children by advisory teachers of the deaf visiting as infrequently as twice each term and as often as once a day, in five cases where hearing losses were in excess of 90 dB (*see* chapter 5). Similar percentages have been found in the education authority of Hereford and Worcester in South Yorkshire and Cornwall and at the Shepherd Centre for Integrated Deaf Education, University of Sydney (Australia) and in New Zealand (personal communications from E.W. Stanton, Mrs A. Alderton, Mrs A. Shepherd and M.B. Parsons). In northern Italy, by 1981, the proportion of individually integrated children who were sufficiently deaf to wear hearing aids, was no less than 96 per cent (*see* chapter 4), in contrast to United Kingdom averages of 44 per cent segregated or semi-segregated and 54 per cent individually integrated (in 1976).

Useful data was obtained recently in a survey made by the Commission of the European Community (Medical)[152] of all the children in eight countries who were born in 1969, were eight years old or more, and had mean better ear thresholds of 50 dB or more. It was found that no less than 98.2 per cent of these children in West Germany attended schools for the deaf, while in Italy, fewer than 40 per cent did so (and, as indicated above, only 4 per cent in northern Italy). (*See* Fig. 1.)

Not all integration programmes work effectively, however, and examples

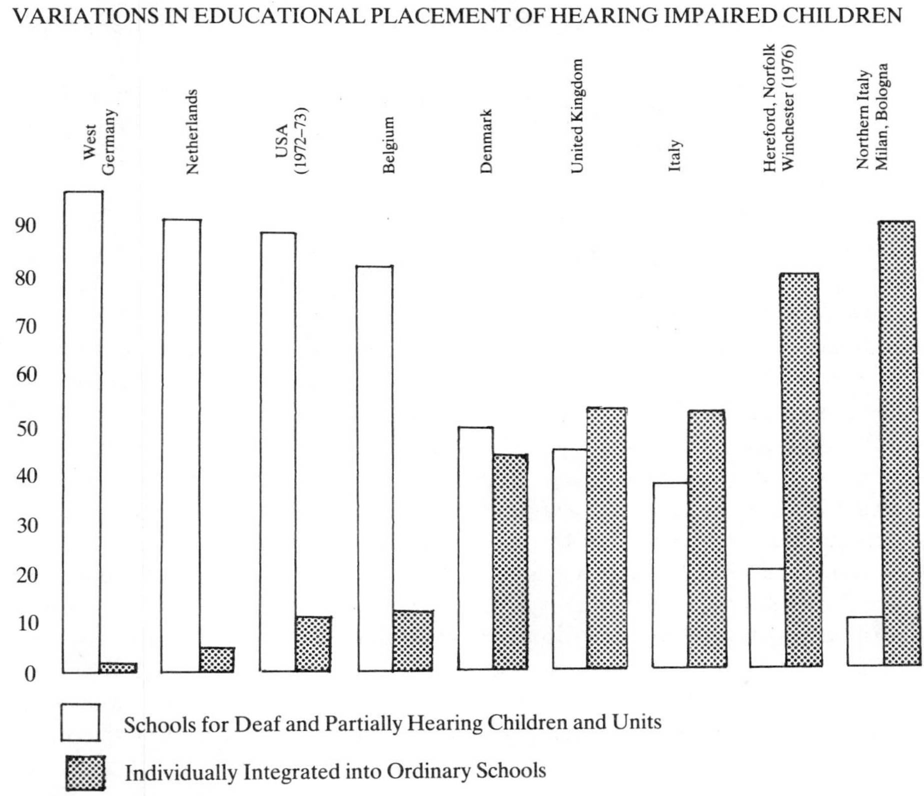

Figure 1 Variations in educational placement of hearing impaired children.

are given later of some of the quite serious difficulties which can occur. However, many of these problems have arisen through factors such as lack of planning, faulty diagnoses of children's problems, lack of personnel and inadequate or non-existent training of teachers, parents and welfare assistants.

Emphases on *individual* educational treatment

In a recent report from the Carnegie Foundation in New York, the point was made that, in the Western world, we had got past the stage of 'education for *all*' and were now concerned with 'education for *each*'. William C. Healey, the Director of School Affairs in the American Speech and Hearing Association, observed that Dr V.V. Yater in her book, *Mainstreaming of Children with a Hearing Loss*, suggested that 'integrated education should be pursued with a commitment and competence that will help to break education's moratorium on *individual* learning.'[236]

Useful descriptions and arguments in favour of informal but orderly methods of teaching rather than the more formal, traditional ones were given in chapter 19 of the 1966 *Report of the Central Advisory Council for Education*

(*England*) *on Children and their Primary Schools* (the Plowden Report). The committee suggested that modern primary schools in England had either adopted or were moving towards this approach.[178] This greater emphasis on *individualisation*, it said (chapter 21), was extremely helpful to children with special needs, and a less authoritarian approach in a number of secondary schools would be welcomed.[42] Subsequent Department of Education and Science reports have also emphasised the value of individual treatment for all children and particularly for those with special educational needs.[73,74,75,80,82]

Sir Alec Clegg stressed the importance of catering for individual needs in ordinary schools during an address at the centenary celebrations of the Education Act of 1870 at the Central Hall, Westminster on 1 May 1970.[41] He observed that 'many junior [primary] schools were leading instead of following society in making learning an exciting and happy business and ensuring that every child was treated as an individual who mattered.' Sir Alec was not sure that all secondary [high] schools were so aware of the need for individual treatment within the comprehensive school system.

In 1977, Karchmer and Trybus,[130] after conducting a national survey in the United States, observed that integration programmes enrolled 'the highest proportion of children from high-income families'. Brill[22] also considered that one of the elements of success in main-streaming was a great deal of time 'spent by parents working individually with their own children' and making full use of pre-school programmes, speech and hearing clinics and correspondence courses – 'all of which take a great deal of time'.

One factor which has been found to affect the amount of language received and used by deaf children in classrooms is the use of *group* teaching methods rather than *individual* ones.[11,56,108] It is easy to show, for example, that a child who speaks, say, three times during the 15 minutes of a group lesson will speak 25 or more times in five minutes when working with a teacher on the same topic on a one-to-one basis (*see* Table 1). If Professor Pittenger's observation during a practical teaching session, that 'deaf children are only learning language when their lips are moving',[177] is basically valid, then it might (somewhat frivolously) be suggested that the child above, when being taught individually, was in a better learning situation by a factor of about eight to three!

Socially, it has also been found that regular association by one hearing-impaired student with a class of normally hearing ones frequently results in his or her quite warm acceptance into the group.[52,65,235] Fig. 2 illustrates that, where two or more such children are attached to an ordinary class, interaction with normally hearing students is usually very much less.[114] It should also be remembered that the speech and syntax of the ordinary children is, of course, much more normal than that experienced when the deaf child is communicating only with others who are hearing-impaired.[12]

Although it is generally agreed that individualised education has great merit, economics and the availability of trained personnel have both caused problems in providing it for most children. There are today, however, some

Table 1 Oral-response frequencies during group and individual language lessons. Note the large increases in response when Child B, Child D and Child F are worked with individually.

	NUMBER OF CHILDREN IN CLASS	MEAN AGE OF CLASS IN YEARS	AGE OF CHILD	SPONTANEOUS RESPONSES IN 5 MINUTES	EVOKED RESPONSES IN 5 MINUTES	TOTAL
CLASS I *Group teaching* Child A	9	9.3	9.4	6	2	8
Child B	9	9.3	8.7	1	2	3
Individual teaching Child B			8.7	14	13	27
CLASS II *Group teaching* Child C	4	7.6	7.6	4	3	7
Child D	4	7.6	7.2	0	1	1
Individual teaching Child D			7.2	15	10	25
CLASS III *Group teaching* Child E	6	5.5	6.1	3	5	8
Child F	6	5.5	5.5	0	0	0
Individual teaching Child F			5.5	11	10	21

encouraging developments in the Western world at least: class sizes in both ordinary and special schools, for example, have dropped markedly during the last 50 years. Reasons for this include the more rapid production of wealth as a result of automation, the recent drop in the birth rate in nearly all countries, significant improvements in preventive medicine,[234] the proliferation of books, distance education programmes,[70,97,156] audio-visual aids and other attractive teaching apparatus which enable children to work more independently in small groups or individually. As indicated in chapter 8, the saving on transport and building costs and the reduction in the number of non-professional staff currently employed in special schools and units can also reduce costs, thus enabling an increase in the amount of individual teaching available to each handicapped boy or girl.

Another very significant factor in the provision of more individual education for all children, could come from the developments in micro-electronics. By using electronic processors for example, one person is now able to produce all the electric light bulbs required for the whole of Canada. It is not

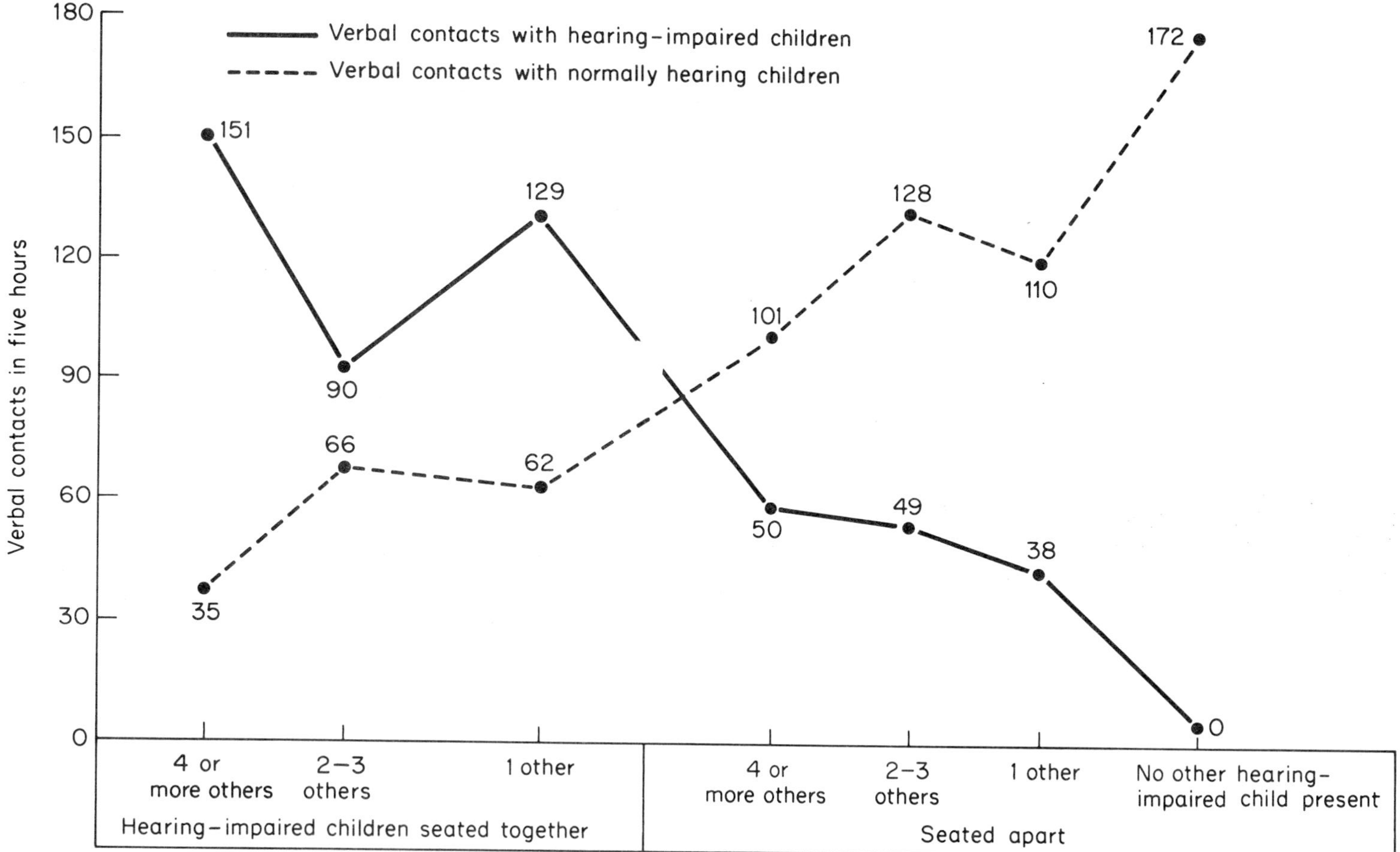

Figure 2 Verbal interaction between a total of 64 hearing impaired children and their normally hearing classmates in various classroom situations in nine ordinary schools (Hemming[114]).

surprising that the developments in micro-electronics since 1948 were described as 'almost as significant as the invention of the wheel' by the Advisory Council for Applied Research and Development (ACARD) in a report to the British Government in September 1978. They are becoming all-pervasive, being able to extend and displace a wide range of intellectual skills, and in consequence represent 'the most influential technology of the twentieth century'.

Professor Stonier of Bradford University suggested, in 1979, that 'the next generation may find that it needs no more than 10 per cent of its labour force to provide it with all the material goods it requires'. This could be highly significant to those concerned with special education since Stonier goes on to suggest that 'the primary activity then will become education, health and social care.' If this comes about, one can predict significant developments in greater individualised treatment both at home and in school, for handicapped children and adults by those freed from routine occupations.

The Warnock Report,[232] after pointing out that one child in five had a significant educational handicap, stressed that the obvious place for the majority of these was in their local ordinary schools. It did not, however, say a great deal (only one page) about *individual* integration for the more seriously handicapped children – those who had traditionally been sent to special schools – and the setting up of units in ordinary schools seemed to be as far as the committee was prepared to go. As will be shown, however, doubts have

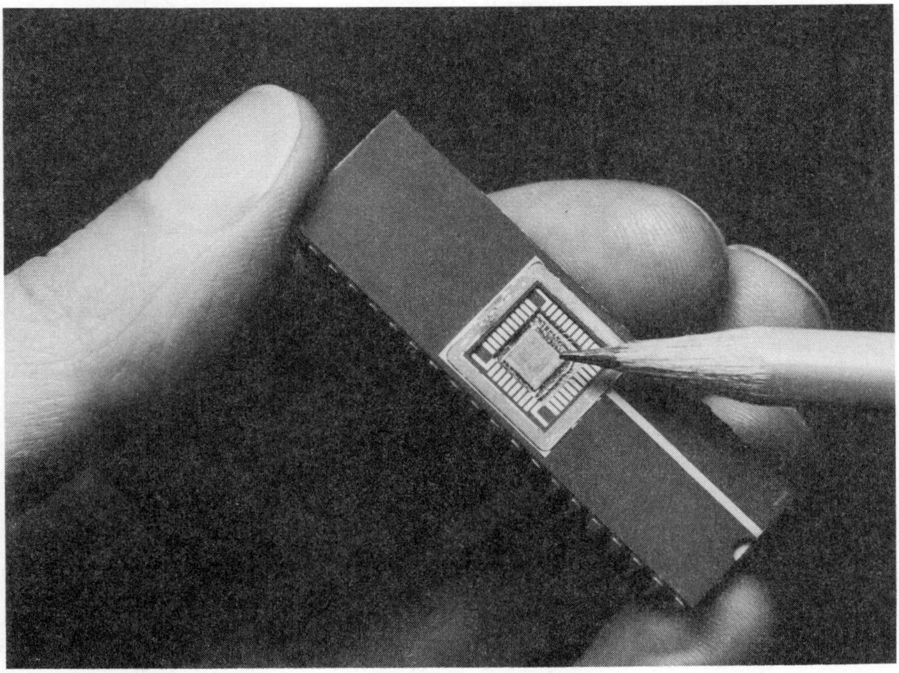

Figure 3 Microprocessors are now carrying out an increasing number of vocational functions previously performed by men and women.
(Photograph: courtesy of Times Newspapers Ltd).

been expressed about the efficacy of units as far as most hearing-impaired and some other handicapped children are concerned.

Arguments for and against segregated day and residential schools

In the past, special schools frequently developed because religious groups and philanthropists felt that some education should be made available to children with special needs. Teachers in ordinary schools felt unable to meet the needs of such seriously handicapped children, or that they were disrupting the work of ordinary boys and girls. In addition, sometimes the homes of the children were unable to cope with them.

Arguments for

Arguments commonly advanced by administrators and staff of special schools to justify their existence have not infrequently included the following:

- Children are managed by experienced and loving staff who understand their problems and take pride in helping them to grow up into happy, healthy and caring young people.
- Since all the children in the school have a particular handicap, they can feel more at ease during school hours.
- Hierarchies of authority, academic achievement and physical activity can develop and many children can experience more success and be given greater responsibility in the most cloistered atmosphere of the special school than is possible in the more competitive conditions of ordinary schools, especially large ones.
- Class sizes are smaller and therefore more individual treatment and more homogeneous groupings are possible.
- In residential schools, good food, proper rest, a daily bath or shower, regular physical exercise and physical check-ups and so on, can significantly improve a number of children's physical health and, as a result, can make them more able to enjoy both educational and social aspects of life. The residential school can be an invaluable 'safety net' for children who, for one reason or another, cannot live in their own homes.
- The modern trend towards weekly boarding for four or five nights each week, rather than full-time residential care, enables a child to receive the best of both worlds.
- Some children can be over-indulged by parents, and attending residential schools where, for example, they have to learn to wait their turn, to share with others, care for younger or less able children, to tidy their bedrooms and iron their clothes, can be good training for them. They also learn to appreciate their homes more.

- ★ There is always company in the special residential school. No child is left alone for hours at a time and he or she can look forward to games and other activities with friends – often in well-laid-out and safe areas with good play apparatus which is not available at home.
- ★ Teachers and hostel staff on duty during 'out-of-school' time can supervise homework and explain, say, television programmes and material found in magazines and books, sometimes better than the child's mother or father.
- ★ The children ultimately go out into life justifiably confident that they can take some useful and satisfying vocation, usually in the open employment field and, in a few cases, in sheltered workshops.
- ★ Some can make and retain friendships with unhandicapped as well as handicapped people – usually marrying and becoming conscientious and very loving mothers and fathers.

Arguments against

True though the above points are in certain cases, there are also numerous contrary arguments to most of them.

Although there are many 'experienced and loving' members of staff in deaf schools, this could not, of course, be said of *all* the staff. Indeed, it is not uncommon to find a proportion of inadequate men and women employed in special schools. A number have found a sanctuary where many of the day-to-day decisions are made for them, where usually all their meals are provided for them, laundry is done, their rooms are cleaned and beds made (sometimes by the children), and comfortable lounges with television sets provided. Apart from innate indolence, a number of staff bring their personal problems with them. When schools are placed in remote country areas, it is frequently difficult to maintain staff, and head teachers and matrons have sometimes commented that they have had little opportunity to obtain *any* staff, let alone select really satisfactory house parents or resident teachers.

Although it has been possible to detect a much greater awareness of handicapped children's needs in residential care during the past, say, 20 years,[219,224,225] much still remains to be achieved in many schools. Courses in administration and in the psychological, emotional, physical and social needs of children should be made obligatory for head teachers, matrons and senior members of staff. One cannot but feel, however, that most of the improvements in residential care of handicapped children are partial steps towards providing satisfying home life for them. One foresees very serious attention being paid in the coming years to parent guidance and support for all families – particularly for those where one or more members are handicapped.

Stereotyping of handicapped children is common when they are all congregated together in one school. Comments by teachers and hostel staff that '*the deaf* can do this' or '*the deaf* are not good at that' are common. The

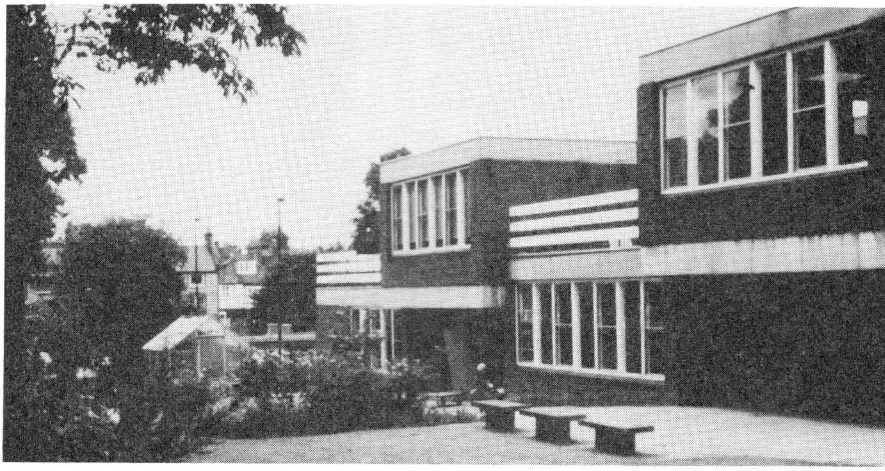

A

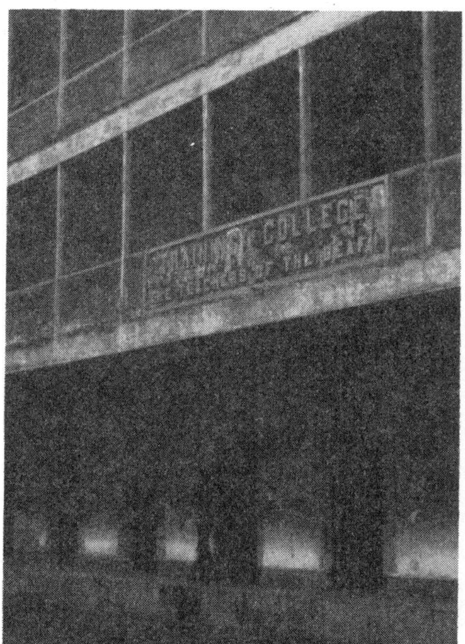

B

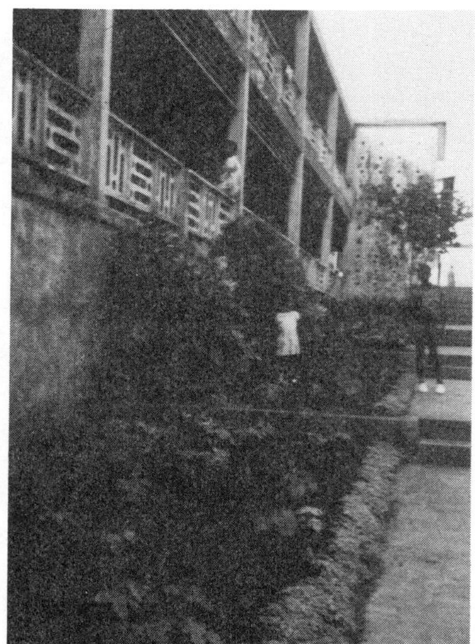

C

children also develop inaccurate views of themselves and of unhandicapped children as a result of being segregated from them. These inaccuracies often (but not, of course, always), result in an over- or under-rating of their own abilities. Over-rating of the abilities of ordinary children can also result in a lack of confidence.

Staff in schools for deaf children frequently try to give them experience 'outside', especially in sport, and success in team or individual events certainly does give the children confidence. One of the very encouraging aspects of enabling these children to be taught in ordinary school classrooms, however, is that they can observe a wide variety of ordinary children closely and can often see that intellectually and socially they are equal to them

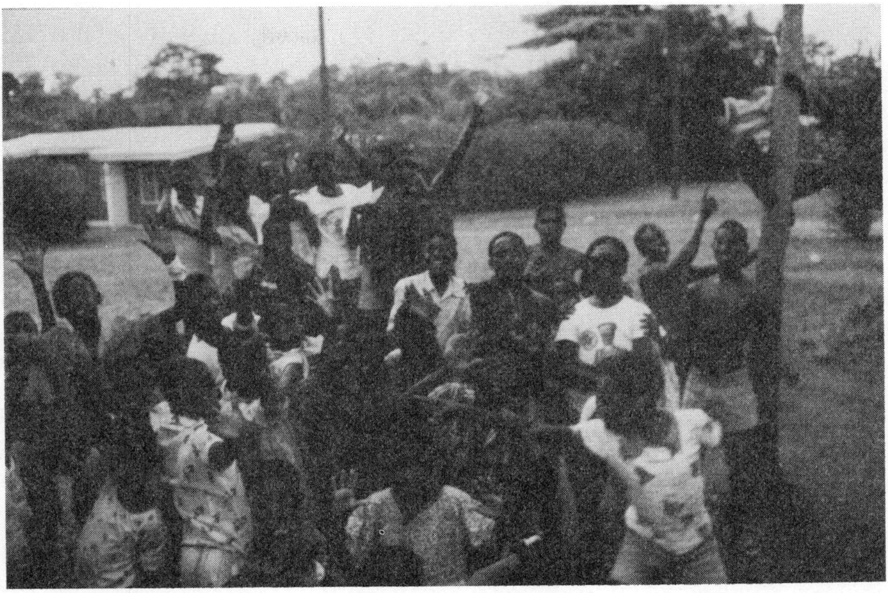

D

Figure 4 Special schools for deaf children in (a) England, (b) India and (c, d) Ghana.

in perhaps all situations except those involving oral language skills. Adjusting daily to a well-ordered, normal environment can only be of benefit to them.

Supporting staff can arrange for a handicapped child to have experience of exercising authority and responsibility in an ordinary school. It might be very modest, of course, for example, seeing that tables are neatly arranged, or that books are put away tidily. More capable children can become class librarians, or responsible for the equipment in the photographic club – there is a host of responsibilities within any school. Some head teachers have adopted the attitude that the school is not '*my* school' but '*our* school': if a window or door is seen to have come off its latch and is banging in the wind, for example, it should be closed by the first person who sees it, rather than he or she feeling that 'that's not my job'.

It has been shown (Table 1) that even in classes of four deaf children, the amount of teacher/pupil interaction can be far less than when the child is managed on an individual basis. With the low reading ages of many of the children in deaf schools and units, it is not possible for a teacher to leave them to work alone for more than short periods while he or she does individual work with each member of the class.

Class size in an ordinary school is, of course, an important consideration when adding a severely handicapped child to it. More important still, however, is adequate and imaginative support teaching.

In Hereford and Worcester, in 1976, 20 per cent of the hearing-impaired children were sent to boarding schools. In every one of these 51 cases, this was due to some serious social or psychological problem at home. (The other

80 per cent were able to attend their local ordinary schools individually, with support from itinerant teachers of the deaf.) When residential care is necessary, it need not be offered in large residential schools. It can often be arranged much nearer the children's homes if organised on the 'cottage home' system,[224] and this is strongly recommended.

Robert Shields, in his recommendations for the residential care of maladjusted children,[201] suggested that to be therapeutically effective the school must reproduce 'as nearly as possible, the good home situation'. He felt that 'only under such conditions can a child establish meaningful relationships with adults' which will parallel those 'of a healthy parent–child relationship'. Dr Shields has concluded, along with many others, that the arrangement best suited to disturbed children (and indeed to the vast majority of those who, for one reason or another must live away from home) is the cottage system. Here a small group of children live together in a house under the care of permanently assigned house-staff. (*See also* Dale[51] [chapter 5], Townsend[225] and Burmeister.[28]) Shields argues strongly for the uninterrupted maintenance of warm child/houseparent relationships. Rota systems, for example, were quoted as responsible for undermining both good relationships between staff and children, and also the personal satisfaction which the staff hoped to gain for themselves.

Children attending boarding schools so that they will appreciate their homes more and learn to be less self-centred are valid points for certain children, for a short period. If these are the *only* reasons, however, even weekly boarding throughout a child's school life is too high an emotional price for most children and parents to be asked to bear. Shorter excursions away from home to Scout or Girl Guide camps are recommended, as are holidays or weekends with loving and capable friends or relatives.

A significant cautionary observation on establishing segregated special educational services was made in 1980 by John Fish,* who was, until 1981, senior staff inspector for special education in the Department of Education and Science. When he was an inspector of special education in an English education authority in the 1960s, just over 100 children in ordinary schools were identified as educationally retarded and needing special educational treatment, and a special school was set up for them. Towards the end of the first year, Mr Fish thought it prudent to write again to all the head teachers of the ordinary schools and enquire whether there were any other children who might not have been identified in the initial survey. To his surprise the number of children listed on this occasion was 101, an almost identical number with that submitted the previous year! He concluded that the teachers had selected the children in their classes who were then most in need of assistance although, of course, they were not so educationally backward as the 100 they had selected the previous year. Rather than set up another special school, it was decided to increase the amount of itinerant and remedial assistance to these teachers and to allow the children to remain in their local

---

* Personal communication from J. R. Fish, October 1980.

schools. Fish's finding was thus similar to that of Professor Dunn in the United States which will be discussed later.

Although most children prefer to live at home, the loneliness of some deaf children when in their own homes can be a very serious problem, especially if they have no brothers or sisters. On several occasions, when bringing their children back to the residential schools in which the writer has lived, parents have made such statements as 'He had his bag packed three days before he was due to come back.' An intelligent girl who left a deaf school, and whose parents then forbade her to associate with other deaf youngsters, became quite morose and truculent at home. Two years later, the head teacher of the school for deaf children, after discussing the situation with the parents, arranged to take her to the local deaf club on one Saturday night. On leaving the club rooms, he asked her if she had enjoyed herself and received the reply, 'That is the first time I have laughed for two years.'

A bright girl (with a hearing loss of 75–80 dB) who, after nine years in a school for deaf children, went to an ordinary high school is quoted in *Deaf Children at Home and at School:*[51]

> Although I was getting a wonderfully satisfying education, I had some personal problems. I ignored them as far as I could, but I couldn't help noticing that I was unable to be completely 'in' with the girls at times. I was reserved and self-conscious of my handicap. When the girls were excited they often talked to one another quickly so I missed some understanding of everyday occurrences. I did not blame them, only at times I wished I was more adaptable with them. At that time, I was terribly shy of boys and remembered not a word spoken to them during three years.
>
> My main aim was to obtain a School Certificate pass to prove to myself and others that a deaf girl could get it if necessary and this I managed to do.

The president of a deaf club, who became profoundly deaf because of meningitis at the age of 12, informed the writer how desperately lonely he had been after leaving the deaf school and becoming apprenticed to a cabinet-making firm. He dreaded Sunday afternoons the most. This highly intelligent man recalled how he had sat in a little shed at the bottom of the garden each Sunday afternoon, too bored and unhappy to draw, to make anything in wood or metal, or 'to do anything at all'. His feelings were of abject misery. A few months later, he was introduced to the local deaf club, met a large number of friendly young people, and said, 'I've never been really lonely since.'

With effective itinerant teachers of the deaf and social worker services, a number of these unfortunate occurrences can be overcome. It is stressed that genuine friendships *have* developed between most individually integrated deaf and normally hearing students (*see* chapters 4, 5, 6 and 7). One must, however, face the fact that severe deafness can impose serious limitations on some people's ability to make lasting relationships with normally hearing children and adults.

Friendships with unhandicapped children are rarely made by deaf children when in segregated schools or even in units in ordinary schools (*see* chapter 3). Friendships with other *deaf* people can, however, be fostered if a child is individually integrated into an ordinary school and appears to need deaf friends. These may be arranged during weekends and holidays, and certainly in adulthood. Pen friends can also be arranged between deaf children who are attending ordinary schools and feel the need to 'talk' to others who are having similar experiences.

Even at Gallaudet College for Deaf Students in Washington D.C., where all staff are encouraged to use both sign language and speech simultaneously, communication can still be a problem. In 1980, a group of 'concerned individuals on campus' which comprised deaf staff members and students, organised a day with the theme 'Communication Unlimited'. Problems identified by these intelligent deaf people included: 'hearing people fear approaching deaf people'; 'not enough deaf people in the "power élite" of Gallaudet College'; lack of awareness of group dynamics on the part of both deaf and hearing individuals; and 'separation between deaf and hearing persons at social functions'.[97]

Introductions to deaf clubs and other informal groups of deaf people should always be kept in mind for those who need them. It is emphasised that, although parents can invite possible friends for their children to parties and outings, help is often appreciated to encourage invitations for the handicapped boy or girl when these are not forthcoming. A brief word about a handicapped person's interests and abilities – as well as any (usually minor) adjustments necessary in getting along with him or her – can often overcome a host's shyness or diffidence, and can make an enormous difference to the enjoyment of the visit, for all concerned.

Some parents *do* require help in aiding their children with school work and reading. Again, alternatives to residential care for this factor alone would include help from itinerant teachers of the deaf, from 'home assistants' (*see* chapter 8), church volunteers, Girl Guides, Scouts, and paid coaches for various subjects. Where parents are unable to assist their children because they have come from abroad and speak little or no English, it is felt to be most important that they should be encouraged to learn the local language as soon as possible. Community resources can be mobilised to assist in this.

The same interest should be shown in the ordinary schools, by specialist teachers and careers and vocational guidance personnel, as is currently shown in some of the day and residential special schools and increasing attention should also be directed to careers and to life after school days are over.[56]

The effect of individual-integration programmes on special schools and classes

The effect that well-organised individual-integration programmes will have on special schools and units can be clearly seen. Day schools for deaf children, for example, are particularly threatened. The majority of the children can be individually integrated into their local schools with varying degrees of support, and the most handicapped can be managed in units in ordinary schools. In north London and Leicester, for example, three and two units respectively now cater for these children, and the remainder attend their local schools individually; the day schools for deaf children have been phased out completely. Residential schools for deaf children, although becoming extremely expensive, still serve a valuable role for those who are unable to live in their own homes. If more well-staffed 'cottage home' facilities are set up, then residential schools, too, may well find themselves more and more short of children.[224]

In the early 1960s it was suggested that the role of the school for deaf children should change.[54] The school was envisaged as a centre where a nucleus of boarding- and day-school children would attend, but also where services 'outside' - at the pre-school unit in the ordinary school, and itinerant teacher levels - would be administered. In a few areas of England and other countries, such a comprehensive service exists. It is interesting that the Warnock Report[232] also envisaged a more varied and outward-looking role for special schools - not necessarily on the administrative aspects, but in making their expertise available to teachers and children with special needs, in ordinary schools.

In this introductory chapter, some reasons for the current trend away from segregated special schools have been advanced. Before individual integration programmes for the more severely handicapped children developed, however, there were the special classes (or 'units') in ordinary schools, and these are considered next.

2

Units and resource rooms: advantages and disadvantages

In the United States, the first special classes for educationally mentally retarded children were established in 1896 in ordinary schools in Providence, Rhode Island. These classes were felt to be, for many children, a better alternative than the previous policy of institutional placement. The controversies regarding such special classes were soon evident, however, and many of them have persisted to the present day. Common criticisms related to the rejection of the handicapped children by their unhandicapped peers, with a consequent loss of self-esteem, and to poor educational results, lack of individual treatment in most units due to the continual demands of other children on the class teacher's time, and the fact that children with other educational handicaps than the one for which the unit had been established had been admitted. This was particularly so in relation to children from ethnic minority groups and those from low socio-economic backgrounds.

Danish teachers were also early in the field of educating their handicapped children in ordinary schools. Special classes were set up in ordinary schools for educationally handicapped children in 1901, and in 1937 all primary and lower secondary schools in Denmark were required conditionally, and by 1958 unconditionally, to give special teaching to children who could not benefit from ordinary lessons.

It is particularly interesting, and significant, that virtually all the blind and partially sighted children who were of average or above intelligence were educated in ordinary classes. The Danish Department of Education indicated that supplies of teaching aids were available from the Braille printing works and from the centres for teaching aids, so that 'blind children may be taught in ordinary classes *without causing serious problems*' (italics mine). At an international gathering in 1972 to discuss integration,[129] the principal of the national school for blind children in Denmark stated that he had sent 40 per cent of his enrolment back to their local schools which had support, 'and this is only the beginning'.

It is a matter for concern that educators of blind children in most other countries have been much less positive in their approach to this question. An excellent study of blind and partially sighted children in ordinary schools in England and Wales was published in 1977.[123] Jamieson *et al.* concluded that more carefully prepared schemes of integration should take place and regretted the bitterness which had not infrequently developed between special schools for blind children and the integrated services in ordinary schools.

In 1968, Professor L.M. Dunn[86] asked, in the journal *Exceptional Children*, whether much special educational provision was justified. As a result of research evidence, he asked whether children with mild mental retardation, and often ethnic minority children with low socio-economic status, had not been wrongly placed in special classes. He also suggested that special educationists had done far too little to develop alternative strategies to help these children outside special classes. Three years later, D.L. MacMillan asked whether one single article had ever had such an impact on the field of special education.[155] R.H. Bruininks and J.E. Rynders[26] have indicated that many of the arguments of authors who felt that special classes were inappropriate for borderline mentally retarded children might be equally applicable to the problems of providing services to the more severely handicapped children.

C. Cope and E.M. Anderson[48] studied English children who had been transferred from a special school for the physically handicapped to units in ordinary schools. Only three of the 55 children were able to attend their local schools, and the remainder were transported for an average journey of 38.7 minutes to and from school (range, 10 minutes to 1½ hours). Not surprisingly, 'virtually no children from either the units or special school named one or more friends from school as those with whom they "usually" played at home'. (Over 50 per cent of the non-handicapped did, however, name one or more friends apart from siblings.)

Forty per cent of the parents in this study regarded the unit placement as special school rather than ordinary school. 'The main reason for some parents viewing the units as "special" was the fact that nearly all of the children were still transported out of their neighbourhood for their schooling.' Thirty per cent of the parents mentioned some aspect of their child's placement about which they were worried, and a number of these points reflected their unease about unit teaching, lack of stimulation, insufficient integration into ordinary classes and excessive travelling times.

Twenty-six of these research children had at an earlier period attended their local ordinary schools. The reasons for their transfer to special schools or units might, in nearly every case, have been overcome if sufficient support from itinerant teachers, physiotherapists and full- or part-time welfare assistants had been provided.

In view of the criticisms of unit placement reported here and later, it is of some concern that Cope and Anderson felt justified in recommending units so strongly as alternatives to special school placement, and gave almost no consideration to well-supported individual programmes.

An indication of the care which should be excercised when managing children with learning difficulties is also given in these extracts from interviews conducted by J. James, a remedial teacher, with two boys who had left secondary schools unable to read adequately.[121]

> *Paul, you told me once that in the first ten minutes of being at secondary school you had what you described then as 'a slap in the face' as far as your ability was concerned. Could you tell me about that again?*
>
> PAUL: That was the calling out of names to go to our new classes. We were all in the hall together. I was put into a special class.* I felt sort of 'branded' right from the first day.
>
> *How did you know it was a 'special class'? Was it explained to you?*
>
> PAUL: No, you could just tell by the people who were in it from the school before. Our names were read out first before all the others, so everyone knew we were 'special class'. I was in that class for a year. We did sort of normal work but with one teacher most of the time so she knew what we were like.
>
> *Can you remember anything that was done in class that really frustrated you?*
>
> CHRIS: If a teacher was explaining something and a few bright kids got it, he just carried on and forgot about the others. It was as if you weren't there.
>
> *If the teacher had asked whether everyone had understood, would you have put your hand up and said 'No'?*
>
> CHRIS: If three or four others had, it would have been OK, but if no one else did, you wouldn't. I remember one time when I told a teacher quietly that I didn't understand something. I thought he'd just go over it with me, but he stopped the whole class and said, 'Chris wasn't listening yesterday so we'll go over this again to make sure . . .'

A 12-week remedial reading programme was developed in Denmark in the 1970s. Psychologist A. Poulson stated that the 'segregation of children with handicaps into special classes came under increasing educational and psychological criticism'.[180] It was stressed that 'children with handicaps should be taught in such a way that they would not be excluded from their normal class community'. Remedial classes were abolished and, instead, reading 'clinics' in each school offered every child as many special reading lessons as he or she required each week – the resources room principle. Although both children and parents were pleased with the change, it was felt that more intensive sessions were required. In the district of Hørsholm in the north of Copenhagen, therefore, an intensive, individualised and systematic reading programme was developed. The course lasted 12 weeks and consisted of 20 lessons each week, three to four of which were devoted to mathematics to ensure that this subject was not neglected. Two teachers with special training in remedial reading managed four children as they took these courses. Four daily sessions were conducted between 8.00–12.00 or 9.00 a.m.–1.00 p.m. each day. All lessons were conducted in one room where equipment

---

* A 'difficulties class' at this unstreamed school for those who had experienced difficulty with school work in previous schools. This class was disbanded the following year.

was set up, and the children were able to rejoin their fellow classmates each day at breaks and for some school subjects.

Positive evalutions were also achieved by 30 former participants of these types of courses, when they were interviewed. Finally, the spirit of co-operation that had developed through the programme led to a far greater degree of rapport between classroom teachers and parents, and also resulted in many of the children being able to make positive evaluations of themselves – thus, the courses not only aided the children educationally, but helped them to develop into happier human beings. One is reminded of F.J. Schonell's finding in 1942, that:

> There is undeniable evidence in nearly every case that adequate and sympathetic consideration of a pupil's scholastic problem is followed by a distinct personality change, not only of individual adjustment in confidence and initiative, but also of social adjustment in his attitude towards his fellows and his teachers.[200]

Units for hearing-impaired children

The first unit for deaf children appears to have been opened in Bayreuth in 1821.[105,144] Many more were established throughout Germany during the second quarter of the nineteenth century, and a number of severely deaf children were enrolled individually in ordinary classes. (Friedrich Moritz Hill,[2] one of the most famous German teachers of the deaf, taught deaf children in a unit attached to the teacher training college at Weissenfels.) Löwe has observed that 'because children of different ages, abilities and degrees of hearing loss were admitted to the unit classes, the task of the teachers of the deaf became impossible. One after the other, all these unit classes were absorbed into the schools for deaf children.'[144]

In the United States in 1965, a report was presented to the Secretary for Health, Education and Welfare by his Advisory Committee on the Education of the Deaf which made some unfavourable comments on a number of the main-streamed programmes that the committee had observed.[187] 'Integration,' the report said, 'seemed more imaginary than real,' and that although the children shared lunch halls and playing areas, there was next to no social contact: '... there appeared to be a *glass wall* between the two groups.'

A survey of 74 of the 162 unit classes for hearing-impaired children in Great Britain was presented in 1967 by two of Her Majesty's inspectors of schools and two medical officers.[81] They observed that 'in the early days it was thought that segregation was an essential factor in the education of deaf children. They were withdrawn from the ordinary schools and brought together in large residential establishments.' The report emphasised that much confusion existed in the use of the term 'unit'. They therefore defined a unit as:

> a group of partially hearing children which is being educated in any one school which also has children of normal hearing, and is under the care of

> one or more teachers of the deaf appointed for this purpose. A *unit* may consist of one class, several classes or a number of individual pupils distributed amongst the ordinary classes, who return to the special teacher for tutorial periods.

Seven different types of unit were identified in this survey, from a single class with the teacher working in complete isolation away from colleagues to some under the authority of the head teacher of a school for deaf children.

In their general observations and recommendations (pp. 45–50), the following were emphasised: careful selection of children for admission; more intensive help for the more severely disabled; regular meetings of unit teachers; avoiding too wide an age and ability range among the children; regular servicing of hearing aids; stable staffing with guidance given to inexperienced teachers; and, finally, the possibility of groups of children with slight hearing losses being taught by ordinary school teachers after the early primary school stage.

Three south of England units 1970–1

In 1970, another study was made of 64 severely deaf children in three units in the south of England, by Iona Hemmings and the writer.[65] The ages ranged from five to 15 years and any child with a gross secondary handicap was excluded. It was hoped to ascertain whether it was possible to teach severely deaf children in units in ordinary schools (Group 1), as effectively as a group of 62 children in two day schools for the deaf (Group 2).

Due to variables such as intelligence, home background, class size, amount of pre-school training and degree of teacher training and experience, it was not possible to compare the educational attainments of Groups 1 and 2. The results obtained for all the children, however, gave no cause for complacency: the average reading vocabulary age[108] of the 22 senior children whose chronological ages averaged 13.5 years was under 8.6 years and speech was virtually unintelligible in many of these 22 cases[51] (consonants were only 53.2 per cent intelligible on average, and vowels 33.6 per cent). The quality of teaching was, overall, high. These results are not, of course, at variance with other studies on larger groups of children in both deaf schools and units.[46,79,101,230]

One factor which it was felt was having a detrimental educational effect on the deaf children was that, due largely to their low reading ages, individual work was difficult for class teachers to arrange and numerous 'whole class' lessons had to be conducted. It had been noted, however, as suggested above (Table 1, p. 7), that most hearing-impaired children respond very well to individual teaching.

Another disappointing factor was to observe in these three schools (and in others) that, although the unit children were usually accepted quite casually by the normally hearing boys and girls, *close* friendships between deaf and hearing children developed very rarely indeed. The deaf children tended to make their best friends with other deaf children since they were usually required to spend several hours a day together in one classroom. In the three cases in this study where a deaf child had made a close friendship with a normally hearing one, their homes were several miles apart; in consequence, another life began for these children when they arrived home from school.

The annual cost of educating and transporting a child to a unit or a day school for deaf children in six local education authorities in Greater London in 1971 was £692 (DES Report, HMSO), but the overall cost per child had risen to £2442 by 1977–78 in the Inner London Education Authority (*see* chapter 5).

New Zealand units 1960–5

An interesting type of infant and primary school unit was developed in New Zealand in the 1960s.[51] The usual pattern was for a small (5m × 5m), sound-treated room to be built on to an existing classroom of an ordinary school (*see* Fig. 5). A group of about six deaf and partially hearing children and a teacher of the deaf were then added to the ordinary school class of approximately 25 children.

For language and speech work, news sessions, story telling and, say, the teaching of a new process in mathematics, the hearing-impaired children were taught in their small room. Roughly half of each school day was spent in the large room, and chairs were left there for the deaf children; some care was taken to place them between normally hearing children at these times. Reading and mathematics activities, music and rhythm, art and craft work, nature study, class visits and physical education were all taken with the two groups combined and both teachers working mainly, but not exclusively, with their own groups.

Advantages and disadvantages of units

The *advantages* observed from this type of provision included:

(1) More children were able to live at home rather than be sent away to residential schools for the deaf and partially hearing.

(2) The children seemed quite quickly to become more socially mature – there was less fighting over trivial incidents such as who was first in line when going in to school.

(3) Fewer 'deaf mannerisms' developed, for example, less signing, less gesturing and less gross facial movement when the children spoke.

(4) The teachers of the deaf had excellent opportunities to observe the interests and language of unhandicapped children. One normally hearing five-year-old, for example, when playing with blocks, exclaimed, 'I'm going to put my submarine in the dry dock!' Most teachers of the deaf in such a situation might be tempted to say to their children, 'That's a boat,' 'A lovely boat, isn't it?' and so on.

(5) The teaching of language was easier. When the deaf children could see

A

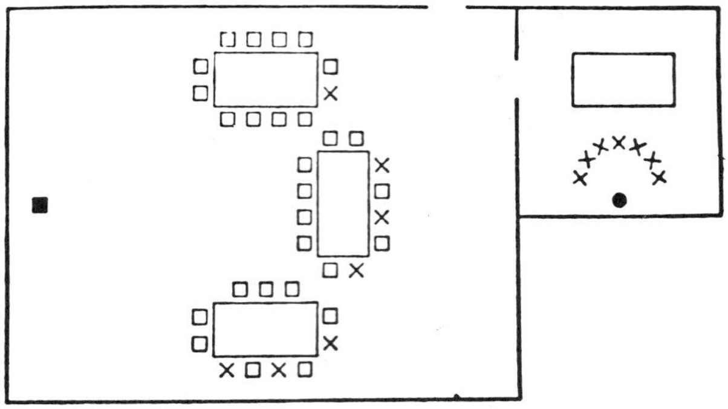

■ Teacher of children with normal hearing
● Teacher of deaf children
× Places for deaf children
□ Places for children with normal hearing

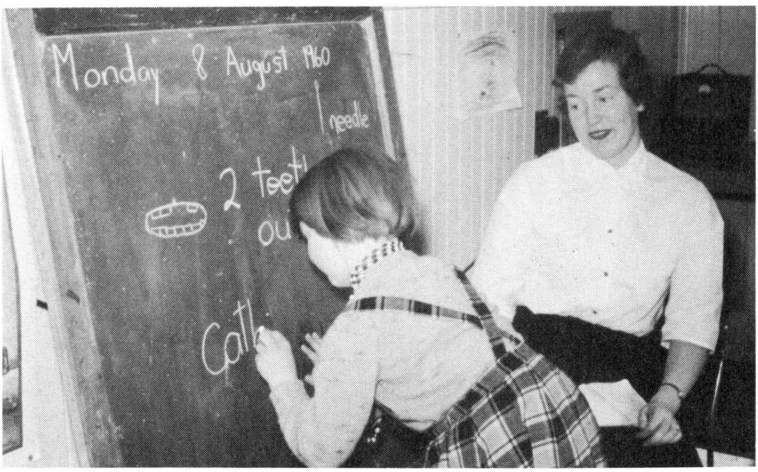

B

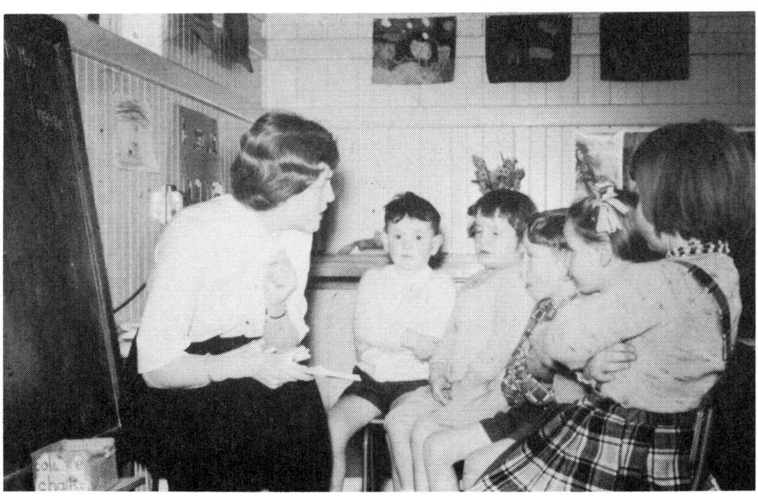

C

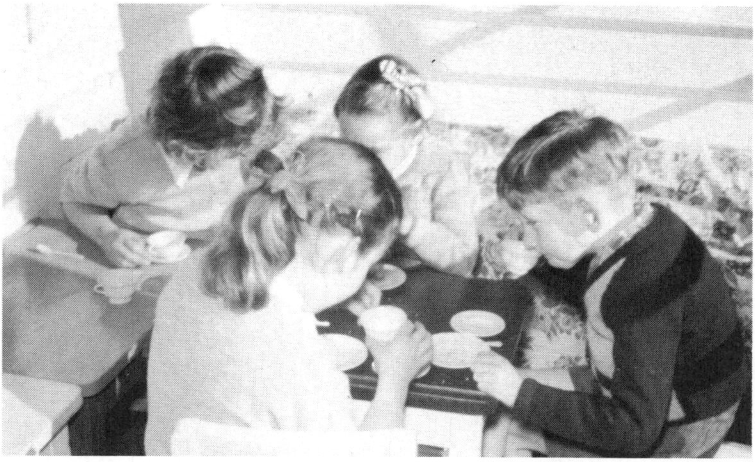

D

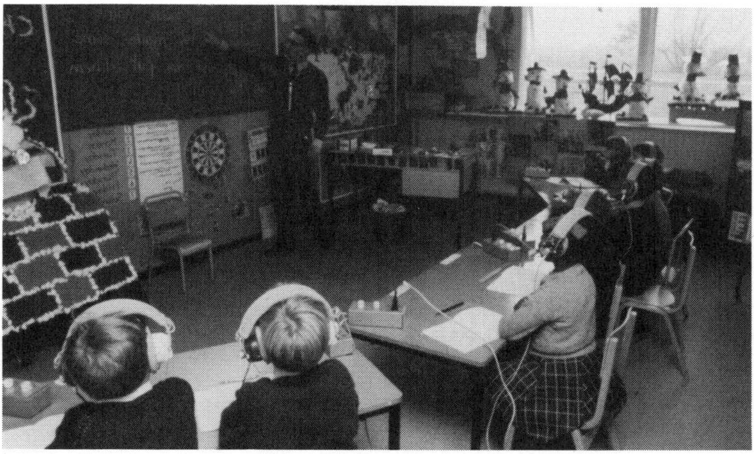

E

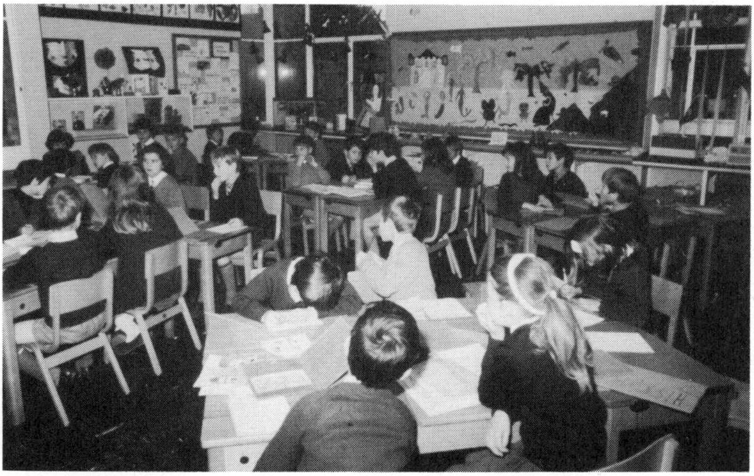

F

Figure 5 Units in ordinary schools developed rapidly in many Western countries during the 1960s and 1970s.

others speaking, reading and writing, they were stimulated to do the same.
(6) Psychologically, it appeared beneficial to both groups. The deaf children could regularly adjust to their handicap each day – realising, for example, that although their language was often impoverished by comparison with normally hearing children, their mathematics, physical education and art work might be very much better. (Intelligent deaf adults have frequently reported having quite serious misconceptions about their capacity to cope in either social or vocational situations after ten or more years in a segregated special school.)
(7) Parents were generally very much happier than when their children were going to segregated special schools. Some said that their friends now realised that their child couldn't be so badly handicapped if he or she was able to attend a unit in an ordinary school.
(8) In 1964, all but three of the 58 children from the Auckland Deaf School area said that they much preferred the ordinary school. In addition to finding their new schools full of interest, it appeared that they felt more normal than had been possible when they were either living in residence at the deaf school or being bussed and taxied to it daily.

The *disadvantages* of unit or resource room provision included:
(1) The heterogeneity of unit classes – groups with wide age, ability and aptitude ranges can, of course, be extremely difficult if not impossible for one teacher to teach effectively.
(2) The disappointing academic achievements of unit children reported in succeeding chapters of this book and elsewhere.[46,52,81]
(3) The difficulties which can occur during the absence of teachers of the deaf or of securing replacements when vacancies occur – especially in more remote areas.
(4) The cost of travel to units or resource centres.
(5) The length of time spent by some children in travelling to and from school. Travel commitments also preclude many deaf children from joining clubs or sports groups which are conducted after school each afternoon.
(6) The isolation from colleagues of the specialist teacher in a single unit class or resource centre.
(7) The lack of sophisticated electrical equipment which large special schools can afford for music and speech work.
(8) The insufficient support to enable regular individual teaching sessions for each child.
(9) Friendships between deaf and normally hearing children are often difficult to make and when they are made are often difficult to sustain due to the distances between the children's homes.[96]
Such disadvantages suggest that this quite expensive type of provision should now be contemplated only after serious consideration has been given to individually integrated alternatives.[86]

Resource rooms

As a means of overcoming the negative effects of many special classes, the concept of the 'resource room' was developed.[157] Handicapped children are enrolled in ordinary classes, but resource teachers assume direct responsibility for some daily instruction of the children in the areas of their special educational needs. In addition, they assist the handicapped children's classroom teacher in planning appropriate educational experiences. The virtue of most resource room schemes is that children with learning problems remain in their own local schools; they are members of ordinary classes, and are withdrawn to the resource rooms at convenient times for additional assistance.

Support or remedial teachers have been increasingly employed throughout Australia since 1970. Brian Courtney, a regional director in Western Australia, in a most useful study,[49] identified 11 extensions to the schools' earlier functions as a result of the increased use of support teachers. Those particularly applicable in the case of handicapped children included: small group instruction (usually within the classroom); intensive re-teaching (often taken by the class teacher while the remedial teacher taught the remainder of the class); co-operative team teaching; release of classroom teachers, sometimes to teach the handicapped child but also, occasionally, to interview parents of a child with special needs; assistance with excursions, visits, camps, and so on; and, finally, remedial teachers as teacher-librarian-teaching aids specialists.

At one primary school in the Australian study, some children requiring remedial help went to the support teacher in the resource centre before school each morning to be helped with problems. It will be seen in chapter 6 that this technique was also observed with individually integrated deaf children in some secondary schools in Auckland and was commented upon very favourably there by teachers, parents and children.

3

Studies of individual treatment

It is interesting – although, perhaps, not surprising – that, in the Western world, the first 20 or so references to educating deaf children describe the use of *individual* methods.[2,127] It was only after the potential of these cases was publicised that agitation began for the education of *all* deaf children and the earliest schools were established. Residential and, later, day schools began appearing in eighteenth-century France, Germany and England, and throughout most of the world this type of special school has remained the major means of educating severely deaf children until the present day. Despite this, a number of cases have been documented of deaf students who have been successfully educated outside special schools and the number of these has increased markedly since the 1960s.

Historically, the first reference to educating deaf children in the Western world was in AD 700 when Archbishop John of Hexham (more commonly known as St John of Beverley) successfully encouraged a deaf youth to speak by imitation. In 1954, the Ewings noted that he adopted a modern educational strategy by using an oral approach to language development rather than a written one.[92] It may also be added that because his approach was on a 'one-to-one' basis, it was also in line with the modern individualised technique. This isolated instance, however, seemed to have little effect on the management of deaf children in Northumberland or in England (or anywhere!) during the next thousand years or so and clearly not too much should be made of it.

Numerous other interesting examples of one-to-one teaching are given in Farrar's *Arnold on the Education of the Deaf*.[93]

J.B. Graser

An inspector of schools in Saxony, J.B. Graser published *The Deaf Mute Restored to Society through Lipreading and Speech* in 1829, and in it he asked '... even if these poor people receive traditional instruction [in institutions], are they thereby put on an equal footing with their fellow men?' His answer, when considered with the most modern thinking today, is, initially at least, quite astounding:

> The state of affairs must come where every schoolmaster is able to teach deaf mutes, and where therefore every school may also be a school for deaf mutes; where every deaf child receives his education in his home town and in the circle of his family; and – it must come to this – that the deaf child should learn the language of his fellows, and mix with them as other hearing people do ... When this has been achieved, one can say that the desired cure has been granted to the deaf child, and the expensive deaf mute institutes are used to the advantage of other pressing school needs.[105]

In the light of all that follows in Graser's book, one must interpret this solely as a basis for his advocacy of teaching deaf children not only language, but also speech (instead of a sign system), rather than as a conscious advocacy of integration, the problems of which he did not consider in this book at all.

Apparently no teacher could be bothered to use Graser's scheme of teaching towards the goal of lipreading and speech, so he did it himself with one boy (no details given) and got him speaking intelligibly and writing to dictation. Royal approval followed and also a command to put his scheme into writing, for closer examination. In his 'Second Preface', Graser expressed disappointment at the continuing general belief in a specialised art of deaf teaching to which only a few may be initiated, therefore excluding hundreds of children from the chance to learn. 'But soon', he said, 'every ordinary school teacher emerging from my training college will be a trained teacher of the deaf, too, and what's more, parents will be teaching speech to pre-school children.'[105]

A. Löwe[138] has observed that, due to poor organisation and the admission to the new units of children of widely different ages, abilities and degrees of deafness, the units were gradually closed. The children formerly in the units were admitted to special schools and there, it would appear, this type of child has remained until the present day (Fig. 1).

Helen Keller and Anne Sullivan

At the age of twenty months, Helen Keller became deaf and blind, and five years later her first teacher, Anne Mansfield Sullivan, was engaged to begin her education.[133] Helen Keller, who died in 1959, became the most celebrated deaf-blind person ever to be educated, and Miss Sullivan's account of her natural, *individual* teaching methods are still so relevant today that they are quoted at some length here.

Anne Sullivan's story of the day, after one month's teaching, when Helen realised that everything had a name is, of course, now a classic piece of writing in the field of special education – and perhaps in literature generally.

> ... We went out to the pump-house, and I made Helen hold her mug under the spout while I pumped. As the cold water gushed forth, filling

> the mug, I spelled 'w-a-t-e-r' in Helen's free hand. The word coming so close upon the sensation of cold water rushing over her hand seemed to startle her. She dropped the mug and stood as one transfixed. A new light came into her face. She spelled 'water' several times. Then she dropped on the ground and asked for its name and pointed to the pump and the trellis and suddenly turning round she asked for my name. I spelled 'Teacher'. All the way back to the house she was highly excited, and learned the name of every object she touched, so that in a few hours she had added 30 new words to her vocabulary. Here are some of them: door, open, shut, give, go, come – and a great many more.
>
> P.S. I didn't finish my letter in time to get it posted last night; so I shall add a line. Helen got up this morning like a radiant fairy. She has flitted from object to object, asking the name of everything and kissing me for very gladness. Last night when I got in bed, she stole into my arms of her own accord, and kissed me for the first time, and I thought my heart would burst, so full was it of joy.

Five weeks later, Anne Sullivan wrote:

> We have begun to take long walks every morning, immediately after breakfast. The weather is fine, and the air is full of the scent of strawberries. Our objective point is Keller's Landing, on the Tennessee, about two miles distant. We never know how we get there, or where we are at a given moment; but that only adds to our enjoyment, especially when everything is new and strange. Indeed, I feel as if I had never seen anything until now, Helen finds so much to ask about along the way. We chase butterflies, and sometimes catch one. Then we sit down under a tree, or in the shade of a bush, and talk about it. Afterwards, if it has survived the lesson, we let it go; but usually its life and beauty are sacrificed on the altar of learning, though in another sense it lives forever; for has it not been transformed into living thoughts? It is wonderful how words generate ideas! Every new word Helen learns seems to carry with it necessity for many more. Her mind grows through its ceaseless activity.

As a result of this child-centred, individual approach, Anne Sullivan was able to teach her grossly handicapped (though highly intelligent) pupil no fewer than 625 words in the first five months after the memorable day at the water-pump.[51]

Anne Sullivan found that a *natural* approach was required in teaching Helen language – 'I shall talk into her hand as we talk into the baby's ears.' A month later she observed that 'since I have abandoned the idea of regular lessons, I find that Helen learns much faster.' During the 'first two years of Helen Keller's intellectual life' she required her to 'write very little . . . Too often, I think, children are required to write before they have anything to say. Teach them to think and read and talk without self-repression and they will write because they cannot help it.'

Hundreds of successful teachers of deaf children, such as Irene and Ethel Ewing,[56,91,92] Mildred Groht[106] and Antoine van Uden,[228] have more recently used and recommended this 'natural approach' to language work for teachers of classes of deaf children. Although agreeing with this, the point is emphasised here, and throughout this book, that *individualised* natural methods (as used by Anne Sullivan), can be much more sensitive to each child's needs and interests. They are also much easier to use than group ones and are usually much more effective in aiding a child's acquisition of both language and speech.

Other useful teaching points discovered by Anne Sullivan in her individual work with Helen Keller, which are as relevant to parents and teachers of deaf children in the 1980s as they were 100 years ago, include:

* To find what interested the child most and make that the starting point of the next lesson. 'Never talk to a child about things that are distasteful or wearisome to him.'
* Helen acquired language 'by practice and habit rather than by the study of rules and definitions'. John Macy commented: 'Of grammar Helen knew nothing and she cared nothing for it.'
* It is 'not necessary for a child to understand everything in a book before he can read it with pleasure and profit.'
* One should encourage questions and answer them honestly. 'The question is the door to the child's mind.'
* 'Books are the store houses of knowledge.'

Dr Pierre Gorman

Born in Melbourne, Australia, in 1924, Pierre Gorman was the only child of a French mother and an Australian father, a lawyer who later became a Queen's Counsel.[104] At the age of six months, Pierre was found to have no useful residual hearing so, six months later, his mother took him to Paris looking for help and guidance on his future upbringing. She was fortunate to be introduced to Dr Henriette Hoffer, a gifted medical doctor who previously had been a teacher of deaf children and also possessed a diploma in phonetics from University College, London, where she had studied under the phonetician Dr Daniel Jones. Dr Hoffer advised Pierre's mother to regard him as an ordinary child who could not hear and not as a deaf child.

At the age of six, Pierre was sent to Melbourne Grammar Preparatory School for normally hearing boys – at first for only half of each school day, returning home in the afternoons for special lessons in language, lipreading and speech from his mother and a teacher of deaf children. Gradually he spent more and more time at school until by the age of ten he was staying full-time and the special lessons at home were given after school hours and at the weekends. He remained in the school until 1942; in his final year he was appointed a prefect, was awarded his school colours in rowing, and for the last two years was senior boy in charge of the school library. He also obtained first-class honours in chemistry in the Victorian public school exams.

From 1943 to 1950 he was at the University of Melbourne where he obtained his Bachelor of Agricultural Science, a Diploma in Education with honours, and the Bachelor of Education degree. In 1954 he moved to Corpus Christi College, Cambridge University, where he did research in the social psychology of deafness. He was awarded the Doctorate of Philosophy from Cambridge University for his thesis on 'Certain social and psychological difficulties facing the deaf person in the English community'. Dr Gorman is currently on the research staff of Melbourne University.

Ruth Dolbear

Ruth Dolbear (née Stephen) is another quite remarkable example of a brilliant though profoundly deaf person who received extremely capable support from devoted parents and ordinary school teachers. She minimised her handicap to such an extent that she was able to attend ordinary schools and the University of London, where she took a Bachelor of Dental Surgery degree at King's College without any support from itinerant teachers or special lecturers. Before her marriage, Ruth Stephen practised as a dentist in central and south London.

The following introspections by Ruth Dolbear[208] on her education as she recalls it, contain so many points which are of help to other deaf students and also to parents, teachers and administrators that they are quoted here in considerable detail. It is clear that most of the discomfort and embarrassment that she occasionally was caused could have been avoided if even a *little* individual support from specialist teachers had been available to her each week, from infant school days to the end of her university career. When Mrs Dolbear read of the integration research in north London (chapter 5) with the daily help of teachers of the deaf and support teachers, she wrote (1974): 'Good luck with your experiment. I can see I was born too early! Although I enjoyed my schooling, there were times, especially during ill-lit drama rehearsals, etc., when I remember guessing hopelessly about what was going on.'

> I was born almost completely deaf as a result of German measles, but it was not until I was 18 months old that my deafness was diagnosed. My mother was put in touch with the Department of Education of the Deaf in Manchester where I was seen by the late Lady Irene Ewing. She advised that my schooling should begin when I was two and a half years old. My mother, who had been a science teacher before marriage, decided to take the three-term course for teachers in the education of the deaf in order to teach me herself.
>
> I do not think I fully realised that I was deaf till I was about six. I began to wonder when I saw my friends talking to each other and to adults in a

quick, mumbling way, which was impossible to lipread. That made me feel younger, backward and very humble. I hopefully thought I would catch up somehow and talk like the others. The fact that I did not realise that there was such a thing as *sound* made me sometimes appear impertinent. I did not know that a school bell was rung at the end of a lesson. If the next lesson was swimming, for which I had a great passion, I would put up my hand to remind the teacher to look at the clock!

My mother explained to me that there were many other deaf children and grown-ups. Whenever I felt depressed about it, she would ask me if I would like to go to a school for the deaf where I would not feel 'the only one'. Every time I said no and stopped being depressed. I always had a certain feeling that, from hearing children, I could learn ways of normal behaviour, use of normal facial expressions and articulation, although I could not hear their speech.

When my mother passed her diploma, she began the difficult task of my education and speech training at home. Meanwhile I was sent to a nursery school for three mornings a week. There I began at the age of three to mix with hearing children for the first time.

When I was five, I had to leave the school, but then I was given a marvellous chance when I was allowed to enter the infant class of five-year-olds for art, handwork, gymnastics, swimming and games while I continued to have lessons from my mother. Very often I did not want to go home after one or two lessons. I thought my mother was making me work very hard at home but she only gave me about one-and-a-half hours of lessons daily, as she was very busy with my baby brother, John, and running the home. I did not realise the other girls had lessons at school all day and homework in the evenings. My lessons at school gave me a fine opportunity to do things with hearing girls which, to me, was a wonderful adventure. Of course, this also gave my mother a good break from me.

After many times when I was quietened, I learned to recognise signs when I should stop talking or playing. When a teacher entered a classroom, I saw the other girls stop moving their lips and turning to face the teacher. However, I *still* have a little trouble knowing when I should stop speaking.

Although, on the whole, the girls treated me as one of them, there were times when they made fun of my speech and took advantage of my deafness. I stood up for myself sometimes, but I was hurt. I realised, later on, that I was not the only one being hurt, when I clearly saw girls being unkind to someone fat or someone of a different temperament. At an early age, I knew that life was hard, as well as that there was much kindness.

I was often behind in lessons like French and Latin. I kept looking up in the dictionary during these lessons. I was told to lipread the teacher in class, but I found it such a strain and practically impossible. In spite of a class of 35 girls, the teacher sometimes was able to explain a few facts to me individually.

But I learned mainly from books, blackboard and notes, which I copied from the girl sitting next to me. My mother also helped me in the evenings. [Ruth joined ballet lessons and Girl Guides and enjoyed both.]

Later, I joined the church's youth club, where I met teenage boys. I was painfully shy of them and dared not speak to them in case they should find out my disability. In fact they did not know about it for several weeks. A few of them were kind to me, but they, like me, were too immature and so were not at ease with me.

At school I played in the second and then the first tennis team and also the second hockey team. It always lightened my heart when I was able to carry on a little conversation with a member of the opposing team at the school matches, and I did enjoy visiting the other schools. My deafness was not a great setback, except that I sometimes continued running along the hockey field after the whistle had been blown.

In the sixth form, I wondered what career I should follow. I fancied the idea of a hospital job, as my father often took the family to visit the wards at Christmas. I also wished to work with people rather than with things, because I felt I would like to continue to learn about human nature. My father suggested dentistry. I was very fortunate, because at that time King's College Hospital Dental School offered to show a party of sixth formers around the dental school. There I watched the students treating their patients in the Conservation Department and asking members of staff questions. I felt a great fear at the bottom of my heart, wondering how I could possibly converse with the staff and patients in front of everybody. I decided, however, to take the plunge and apply. I was surprised but delighted when I was interviewed and accepted by the dental school.

After two years in the sixth form, I passed chemistry, physics and zoology at Advanced Level for the University of London General Certificate of Education. But I stayed for another year at school till I was 18, doing scholarship level chemistry and zoology. I was quite relieved, as I did not feel emotionally ready to embark on a university course.

I was most touched when the school voted me to be a prefect. Of course, my duties were rather limited, owing to my handicap, but there were times when I had to reprimand younger girls. Once I went into a classroom to stop a crowd of girls from being too boisterous. I hoped that, when I left them, they were quiet for some time, and that they did not know my legs felt like jelly.

I was both glad and sorry to leave school. I looked forward to starting the first year at King's College of London University. I found the first term exciting, interesting, but also most bewildering! I said to my mother at the end of the term, 'Oh, I'm so glad to have four weeks at home where I'll always be understood.' The students were friendly, but spoke casually to me when I was walking with them along corridors, ascending or descending the numerous stairs. I did not know whether to explain carefully to them about my disability or just nod, grin sheepishly and walk past. The general noise and pushing crowds did not help either. I think I worried too much about being sociable.

Cynthia Menzies

Cynthia Menzies, profoundly deaf with a hearing loss of 105 decibels (dB), spent her early years at home with a governess. She was enrolled from the age of six to 11 in a private school for four normally hearing children taught by a trained teacher of the deaf. In 1970, Cynthia and her younger sister, Katie, were admitted to a small boarding school for girls in Norfolk. A full-time teacher of the deaf was employed to assist Cynthia at various times throughout each school day – helping with school subjects in the classroom or in individual tutoring sessions in a small study (see Table 2). Occasionally one girl ('D') who had poor reading ability accompanied Cynthia to the study room for extra reading help.

When the parents were asked if they would consider three or four other deaf children enrolling in the ordinary school with Cynthia, they were sure that this would not be in their daughter's best interests. They felt, and I now

Table 2 Timetable for a profoundly deaf girl (aged 13 years) in an ordinary boarding school

	MONDAY	TUESDAY	WEDNESDAY	THURSDAY	FRIDAY
9.20	French C+D	French C+D	Study Cookery C	Study C+D	French C+D
10.00	Maths	Religious instruction C	Study Cookery C+D	French C	History
10.40	Geography	Physical education	English	Maths	Maths
11.20			BREAK		
11.40	Games	Art	Science	Needlework	Musical appreciation C
12.20	Religious instruction C	Art	Science	Needlework	English
1.00			LUNCH		
2.30	English	English	Games	English	Religious instruction C
3.10	Science	History	Maths	Games	Singing C
3.50			TEA		
4.15	Geography	Maths	History	Geography	Religious instruction
4.55	Study	Study	Cookery	Study	Study

C: Indicates that the pupil (Cynthia) returns to the tutorial room for individual attention.
C+D: Cynthia plus another member of class requiring remedial reading in tutorial room.

believe rightly, that if other deaf children came to the school with Cynthia, they could be stereotyped and would receive less normal management. Staff would refer to 'the deaf children' as a group – 'The deaf children could come with us on the outing', 'The deaf children are good at art, aren't they?', and 'It won't be much use taking the deaf children to the theatre, will it?' and so on.

After four years at secondary school, Cynthia went on to a college of further education, with a teacher of the deaf assisting two-and-a-half days a week, studying photography and other subjects, and is now working in the photographic field.

Several other people, known to the writer, who were born profoundly deaf have become dentists, psychologists and doctors. In chapter 8 and appendices 7 and 8, examples are given of courses which have been successfully followed by hearing-impaired students in ordinary colleges and universities.

It is hoped that more and more deaf people (and their teachers and parents) will be persuaded to write detailed articles and books about the practical ways that deaf people have found to succeed in their educational and vocational careers and in their lives generally.

A multiply handicapped child

On the Isle of Wight in 1976, a full-time welfare assistant was assigned a five-year-old, profoundly deaf, paraplegic child of very low intelligence. The parents of this child had been advised by two doctors to have her admitted to a mental hospital without delay. The parents and the education authority agreed that this would be necessary ultimately, but thought they would first like to try an integration experiment in the local nursery school where there was a class for hearing-impaired children, and a welfare assistant was provided (at about half the cost of a residential mental hospital placement).

It was possible even for this extremely handicapped little girl to attend a nursery and infant school very happily for three years. Her class fellows enjoyed pushing her in her wheelchair around the classroom, to the lunch hall and elsewhere and the parents reported how happy she was when the mini-bus and her welfare assistant arrived at her home each morning. After some years, the gap between her performance and that of the rest of the class widened and the placement became more and more inappropriate. This was clear to her parents as well as to the welfare assistant and her teachers. She was, therefore, finally admitted to a 'cottage home' type of hospital at the age of eight – coming home to her parents for some weekends and for holidays.

This example illustrates that not *all* handicapped children can be successfully educated in ordinary schools on a full-time basis, nor necessarily throughout the whole of their school lives. In such cases, parents and teachers may have to be prepared to accept partial integration for some children, and complete withdrawal to more suitable segregated facilities at some future time. This limited period of attending an ordinary nursery and infant school and later coming home for holidays and at weekends can bring a great deal of pleasure to these children and comfort to their parents. When carefully arranged, such schemes can also bring pleasure, understanding and satisfaction to teachers and children in the ordinary schools.

PART II

Perspectives from various countries

4

Individualised integration in some developed countries

In various parts of Italy, the United States, Argentina, Canada, Australia, India, the United Kingdom and New Zealand, individual integration programmes for severely and profoundly deaf children have been conducted for a number of years. The ways and means of meeting these deaf children's educational and social needs were often quite dissimilar, and in consequence all are discussed (in some cases very briefly) in this and the three following chapters.

Italy

Some most influential legislation on the education of handicapped children was passed in Italy in 1971. Act 118 stated that: 'Education of handicapped children must take place in ordinary classes in ordinary schools except when the subject suffered from severe intellectual deficiency or from physical handicaps so great that they prevented or rendered very difficult the learning process in the ordinary classroom.'

Since 1971, Dr I.M. Buzzi-Donello, now principal of the Tarra School for Deaf Children, Milan, and her colleagues have established a most interesting individual-integration programme for children who formerly attended, or would have attended, the Tarra School. By March 1980, 96 severely and profoundly deaf children were individually attending their local primary and secondary schools in the city; 17 teachers of the deaf were employed to assist them.

Each primary school child was visited between one and five times each week for periods of up to two hours, depending upon individual needs, with an average of three visits per child per week. Individual tutoring was also offered, usually in the classrooms. In addition, assistance was given to other children in each class after consultation with the class teachers, and this was felt to help the integration of the handicapped child (and of the teachers of the deaf!). New cases were seen by one of the 17 itinerant teachers of the deaf when they were referred from the diagnostic team, and the teacher then decided, with the audiologist and speech therapist, how many sessions each week would be required when each child began attending his or her local school at the age of six.

Italy's Law 517 states that, when a child has been designated 'educationally handicapped' by the medical and psychological team of the local *quartiere*, the class size in the ordinary school to which he or she is attached 'must not exceed 20' (normal classes in Italy have enrolments of 25). This official recognition of the added responsibility of a teacher who deals with a seriously handicapped child in his or her class was very much appreciated by class teachers and itinerant specialists alike.

Head teachers of ordinary schools in Milan also approached the principal of the school for deaf children when they needed individual assistance from the itinerant teachers of the deaf for children with the following disabilities causing language disorders or deficiencies: aphasia, dyslexia, Down's syndrome, cerebral palsy, gross speech articulation defects, cleft palate and, occasionally, for children from non-Italian-speaking homes, or who were socially deprived. In addition, speech therapists in Milan gave guidance to parents of all pre-school hearing-impaired children, assisted them in the *scuola maternale* (kindergarten) between the ages of three and five, and also took responsibility for all children with average hearing losses of less than 70 dB in primary and secondary schools. This, of course, represents a reversal of many of the functions of speech therapists and teachers of the deaf as they exist in the United Kingdom and in most other countries. It appeared, however, to be working out well according to the itinerant teachers of the deaf interviewed.

Dr Buzzi-Donello has drawn up very helpful guidelines for parents, and for teachers of deaf and normally hearing children, which are of assistance when deaf children are transferring from the deaf school to their ordinary neighbourhood school. At the socio-psychological level, for example, she suggested noting the following: an analysis of the child's family situation; any other handicaps; an evaluation of the personality needs of the child; the child's attitude to learning; the child's ability to achieve good relations with teachers and fellow students; the child's behaviour in both study and play situations; and, finally, the degree of acceptance of other children's families.

The teachers of the deaf met at Tarra School each Wednesday afternoon to discuss problems and successes and to obtain assistance from the audiology technician and other colleagues within the school. None of the teachers wished to return permanently to teach in the school for deaf children. When asked why, comments included: 'We don't agree with a segregated policy for deaf children any more', 'It's more interesting', and 'It's much better for the children.'

By 1980, the number attending the school for deaf children had been reduced to only 40 children (from 400 in 1960). It is again highly significant that all but one of the 96 children individually integrated into their local schools (child 3 below) were reported to have established warm relationships with their normally hearing classmates. The school for deaf children catered only for dually and multiply handicapped children, and it was reported that only one new child was to be admitted in September 1980.

By March 1980, the retiring principal of the Tarra School, Dr J. Roda, estimated that approximately 70 per cent of hearing-impaired children in Italy were integrated in ordinary schools. There were, however, wide regional differences. In the north, for example, over 90 per cent were integrated, while in the south the figure was nearer 40 per cent. The region where integration programmes began, and where this approach was currently most widely practised, was Bologna, 50 miles north of Florence.

Parents

Parents were reported to be firmly behind this type of integration programme. The parents of two of the children, who were themselves deaf and had been educated in schools for deaf children, were at first apprehensive about the scheme. When they realised how much assistance their children would receive and how happy their child seemed to be once the project began, they too accepted the project much more cheerfully and could see the benefit of it. (The writer has had many similar experiences with deaf parents in England, New Zealand and the United States.)

Parents were closely involved throughout. Not only were they sent accurate details of work covered each day by the teacher of the deaf or the class teacher, but also meetings of mothers and itinerant teachers of the deaf were held at the school on one afternoon each week. Mothers were expected to attend and nearly all did. (In the rare cases of recalcitrant parents or those who did not take the school seriously, heads of schools – *not* the head of the school for the deaf – arranged to speak to them.) Some parents had work commitments on weekdays, and meetings were therefore arranged on Saturday mornings for them. The week's work for each child was reviewed and parents' problems and successes were discussed. These meetings usually lasted about one hour.

The children

The following are extracts from observations made by the writer during visits made in March 1980 to eight schools in Milan.

Child 1

Aged six years, hearing loss 100 dB. Academic ability above average. Seen daily by the teacher of the deaf. A class lesson was in progress involving the study of good and poor conductors of heat. A jug of hot water was placed on the floor in front of the class (whose tables were arranged in a semi-circle), and wooden, plastic and metal spoons were put into the hot water. The children guessed which spoon handles would be hot and, after taking turns to test the temperatures, they recorded the results in a simple table:

	Scotta (hot)	Non scotta (not hot)
Legno (wood)		√
Plastico (plastic)		√
Metallo (metal)	√	

and these results, with some explanatory sentences and other points – for example, 'We use wood for houses in the mountains because it is a poor conductor' – were to be taken home.

Both the class teacher and teacher of the deaf worked in front of the class, helping each other setting up the apparatus, making blackboard notes, and speaking clearly but animatedly to the class (sometimes both at once!).

The deaf girl and one other were asked by the teacher of the deaf to come out and test the temperatures first. The other children watched and saw clearly how the teacher of the deaf spoke to the deaf child, the problems the child had in understanding and in speaking intelligibly and how the teacher overcame some of these communication difficulties. Such information would inevitably assist the children when they came to talk to this little girl at other times during the day. The atmosphere throughout was purposeful and cheerful; although the handicap was recognised, it was accommodated briskly and not permitted to interfere unduly with the conduct of the lesson.

Child 2

Aged six years, hearing loss 80 dB. Good average ability. Congenitally deaf. Seen by the teacher of the deaf three times a week. Usually taken from class with two friends because the class teacher didn't approve of the teacher of the deaf working in the classroom. Much use was made by the class teacher of well-illustrated handouts for all the children (Appendix 1, pp. 166–7), and although the reading material on these was often felt by the teacher of the deaf to be not quite suitable for the deaf child, the illustrations were helpful and they were useful to take home to the parents. The class were making Easter eggs to take home and all clearly enjoyed the lesson very much.

Child 3

Aged ten years, hearing loss 100 dB. Good average ability. An only child of very intelligent, deaf parents. Three years spent at the school for deaf children and individually integrated for the last two years.

The teacher of the deaf made visits three or four times each week. In this class of 20 children, five had parents who had studied at the university, but the majority had had little education. The deaf child was said to rank about the middle of the class for most subjects. He clearly benefited from the

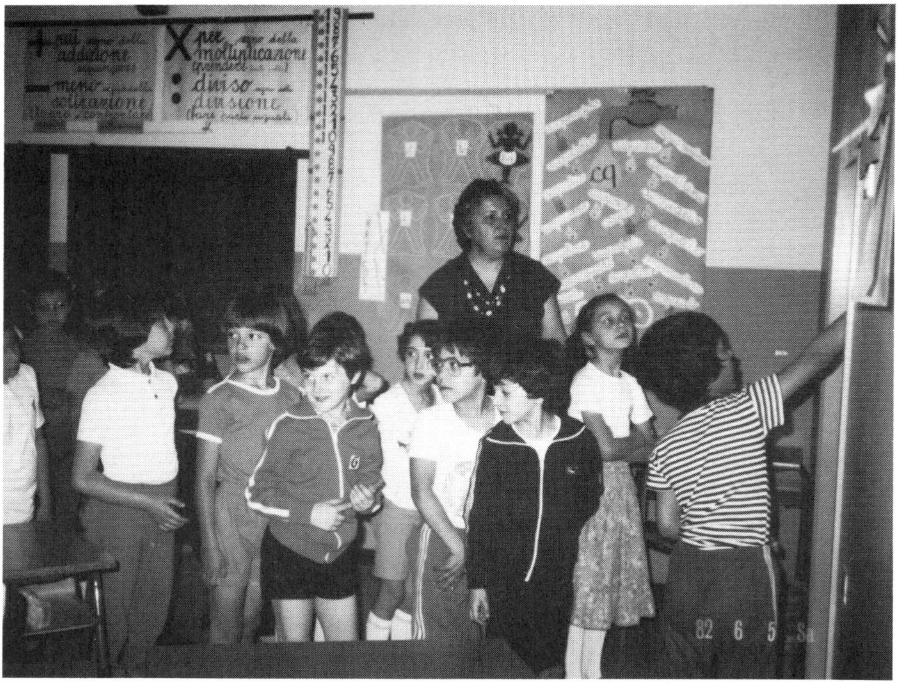
più
addizione
meno
sottrazione
per
moltiplicazione
diviso
divisione
82 6 5 Sa

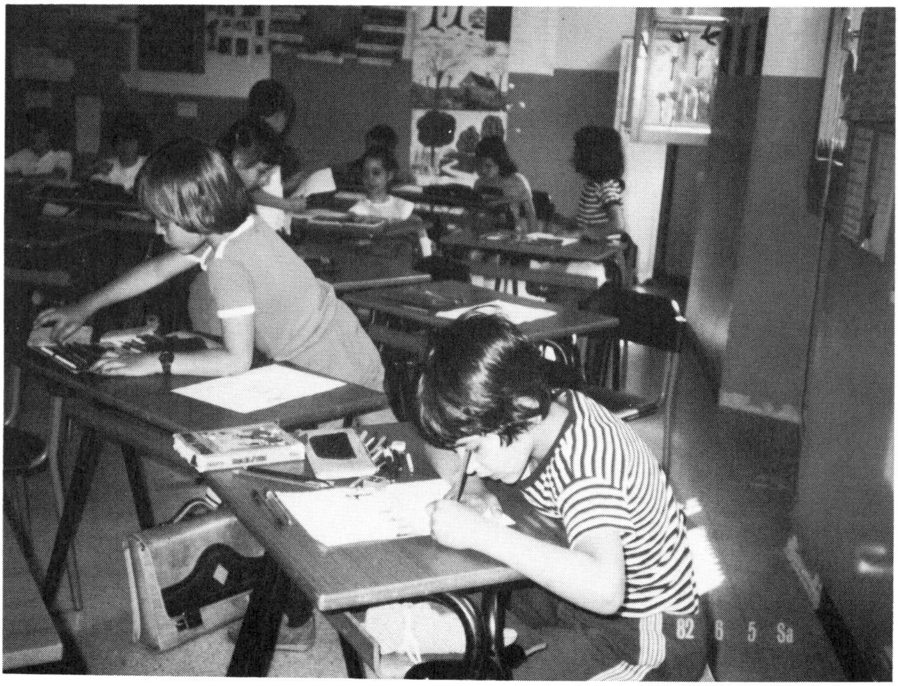
82 6 5 Sa

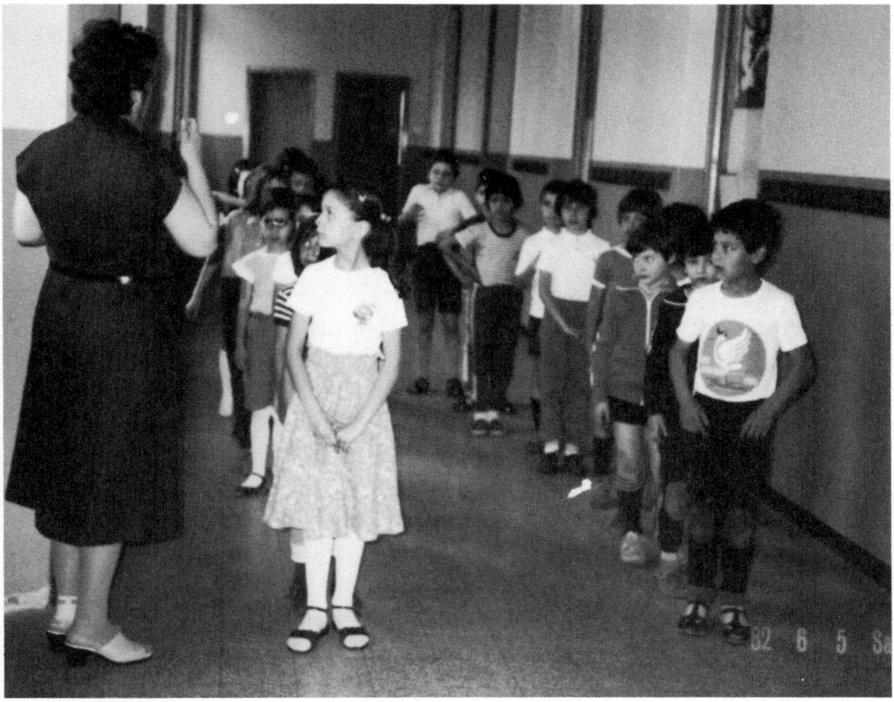

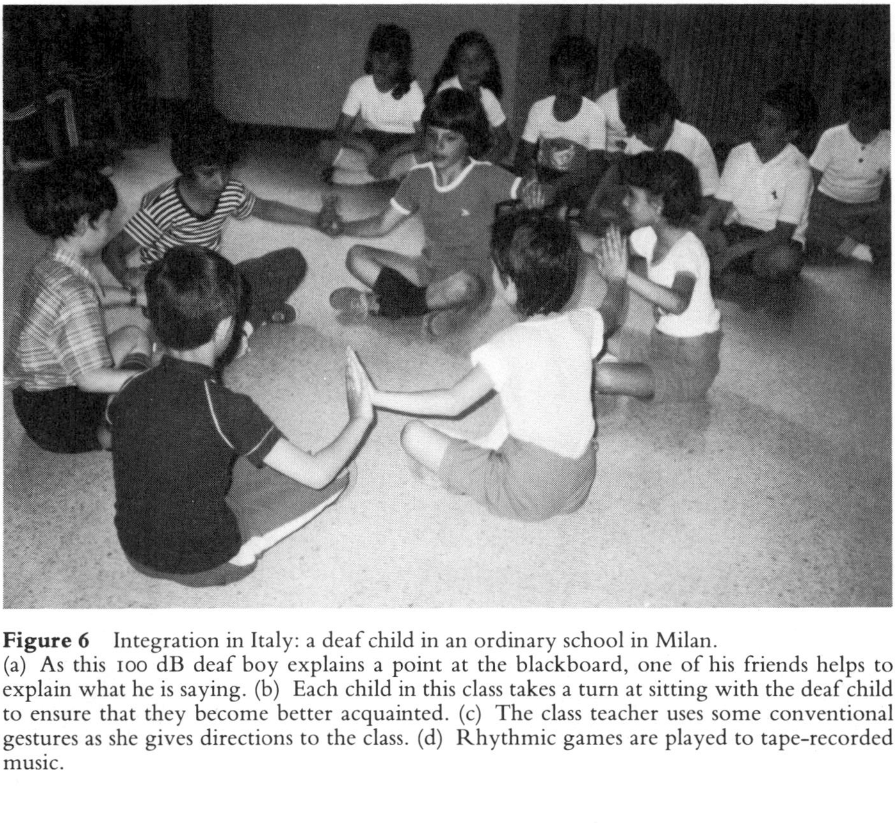

Figure 6 Integration in Italy: a deaf child in an ordinary school in Milan.
(a) As this 100 dB deaf boy explains a point at the blackboard, one of his friends helps to explain what he is saying. (b) Each child in this class takes a turn at sitting with the deaf child to ensure that they become better acquainted. (c) The class teacher uses some conventional gestures as she gives directions to the class. (d) Rhythmic games are played to tape-recorded music.

individual and micro-teaching unit with the teacher of the deaf, although not wanting to be singled out too obviously.

The class teacher found it helpful to the deaf boy, and to a number of the others in the class, if she wrote many of the instructions on the blackboard. She also used the blackboard more in mathematics because 'he doesn't like to be seen being helped too much directly'.

Child 4

Aged ten years, hearing loss 110 dB. Academic ability above average. Aetiology: meningitis at six months. This boy was seen by the itinerant teacher of the deaf for two two-hour sessions each week. Help with school work, and with speech and social adjustment, was given at each visit. Ten minutes of auditory training during each visit was felt to have improved this boy's very intelligible speech, despite his profound deafness. There were 16 children in his class.

The children in the class had been encouraged to repeat statements for this boy. At about seven years of age, he began to 'string words together', and by ten years he spoke fluently, although a little too rapidly. The parents were convinced of the importance of making an early start.

Child 5

Aged seven years, hearing loss 105 dB. Academic ability above average. The itinerant teacher of the deaf saw this little girl for a total of eight hours each week: Day 1 for two hours; Day 2 for four hours and Day 3 for two hours. (During the rest of the week this teacher travelled to other schools and saw: one other severely deaf child; two psychotic children; two with speech problems due to cleft palates; two dyslalic children and one whose speech disorders seemed to be due to mental retardation.)

During the lesson observed, the class, after some lively discussion and acting in which the deaf child was much involved, were asked to cut out five pictures from their workbooks. After these were arranged in the correct order, the children wrote short sentences to make a story, for example:

1 Gianluca is looking at the apples.
2 She shook the tree.

The class teacher assisted each child as required, talking and occasionally writing words or phrases on the blackboard. The stories were taken home to the parents after the pictures had been coloured.

Each Wednesday, during the four-hour visit, the teacher of the deaf met the mother and had a general discussion of events at home and at school, how the previous week's work had been managed and the content of the next week's assignments.

When the class teacher was asked how this profoundly deaf child made herself understood, she said that she could now speak 'fairly clearly'. 'Earlier,' she said, 'she used "body language" and after all, she *is* Italian!' The use of the hands in communication is, of course, a feature of conversations among

Italian people and doubtless accounts for the unusually high proportion of eight-year-old Italian deaf children – 491 out of 668 – who used 'manual' communication in the EEC medical survey of 1977 reported by Martin and Moore.[152] This proportion can be compared to 35 out of 145 in the Netherlands and 109 out of 709 in the United Kingdom.

Child 6

Aged 11 years, hearing loss 95 dB. Aetiology: congenital. Better ear average of 500, 1000 and 2000 Hertz (Hz), although 45 dB at 125 Hz. Excellent speech. Academic ability: average.

This girl had repeated Class 2 and was thus a year older than her classmates. She was seen by itinerant teachers of the deaf for two sessions per week of two hours' duration. On one of these visits, the child worked with the itinerant teacher on conversations, reading, speech and auditory training. Her mother also attended part of this period and was able to ask questions, share information and receive guidance. During the other two-hour period, the teacher of the deaf worked within the classroom on group project work. When asked why these two weekly sessions could not be split into half group or class work and half individual tutoring, the teachers replied that the project work took the full two hours and they felt it best not to interrupt it.

The class teacher commented that she did not feel so anxious now as she had done to begin with, 'because the two of us [teachers] are working together and we are much stronger'.

Secondary school children

By March 1980, 39 secondary schools in the city of Milan had enrolled 57 children (37 boys and 20 girls) who wore hearing aids. A further 22 children attended 19 schools in outer Milan boroughs. Unfortunately, teachers of the deaf were not permitted to teach these children individually in the secondary schools because some of the teachers had not obtained university degrees. In consequence, five teachers of the deaf assisted the most severely deaf of these children by working with them each afternoon when they came into the school for the deaf for tutoring.

An interesting development has been the conduct of classes for secondary school teachers to help them assist the deaf children in their classes. These courses consist of 13 seminars from 3.00–6.00 p.m. on one afternoon each week (Appendix 2, pp. 168–9). Attendance at the classes was optional, but certificates of attendances were given, and when written work was involved, the teachers received credits for this. Six-session courses were also conducted by the school psychologist, dealing with psychological difficulties of children with language disorders.

The overall educational and social achievements of these very deaf children appeared to be very good indeed. It should be noted, however, that they were all of at least average academic ability, and in virtually all cases their parents had been very closely involved in the educational programme.

The United States

In 1961, a study was made by C.D. O'Connor and L.E. Connor of 21 children who had transferred from the Lexington School for Deaf Children in New York City to their local primary or secondary schools.[167] The average age of these children on entering the Lexington School had been 3.5 years; the average length of time spent at this school had been 4.6 years; the average hearing loss was 73.1 dB and the average IQ was 114.6 (on Wechsler Intelligence Scale for Children [WISC], or Merrill-Palmer Scales, or Pintner Paterson Non-Verbal Scales). Class sizes in the ordinary schools ranged from 15 to 54 students with a mean of 19. Ages at the conclusion of this study ranged from six to 19 years with a mean of 13.4 years.

The two authors concluded: 'The results of this intensive study of able former pupils of the Lexington School for the Deaf indicated that about half were unsuccessful in their transfer to integrated classes.' This result with such gifted partially hearing pupils may at first seem to be both disappointing and surprising. When one realises, however, that 35 per cent of the children received *no* extra help once they had enrolled in the ordinary school, and that the other 65 per cent received only occasional visits from a speech or hearing therapist, while guidance personnel, psychologists and remedial teachers were only minimally involved, this would undoubtedly account for much of the reported lack of success. It is surprising that, at the time, the writers did not appear to emphasise this, although in his later studies (see below), Dr Connor certainly has done.[44]

Connor persevered with a variety of programmes to integrate children from the Lexington School into the main-stream, and later wrote that 'between 1968 and 1975 a total of 124 prelingually, profoundly deaf children have been transferred (prior to age 14) to regular school programmes. Only two have returned to a special school as "unsuccessful".' He concluded that the scheme required administrative dedication, teacher-of-the-deaf support and parental co-operation. Dr Connor felt that one of the main factors in the programme's success was the enthusiasm of his own teachers of the deaf, who went into the regular schools to support the children and encourage the ordinary school teachers.

In the most comprehensive survey of the integration of prelingually deaf children in the United States to date, Dr R.G. Brill studied the 12 programmes, each containing at least 30 children, which had reported most involvement with main-streaming.[22] These were selected from data collected by the Office of Demographic Studies at Gallaudet College, Washington, D.C., in the 1975–6 school year. Table 3 (abstracted from two of Brill's tables) indicates that wide variations existed between the 12 programmes in the percentages of severely deaf children enrolled and in the various patterns of integration.

To take one example, Massachusetts Law 877 was passed in that state in 1970 and in many respects resembled the now-famous Education of All Handicapped Children Act, the federal Public Law 94–142 of 1975.[89] Law

Table 3 Number of severely and profoundly prelingually deaf (SPPD) children in each of four patterns of main-streaming in the USA, 1975–6*

	Total enrolment of all children	Total of hearing-imp. (H/I) children	Total SPPD	Pattern 1			Pattern 2			Pattern 3			Pattern 4			Total % Main-streamed
				No. of SPPD	% of H/I	% of SPPD	No. of SPPD	% of H/I	% of SPPD	No. of SPPD	% of H/I	% of SPPD	No. of SPPD	% of H/I	% of SPPD	
Calif: San Diego	117,000	172	129	18	10	14	—	—	—	13	8	10	33	19	26	50
Mass: W. Ross	N/A	126	82	7	6	9	10	8	12	17	14	21	38	30	46	88
Minn: Spec. Dist.	110,292	271	62	14	5	23	48	18	77	—	—	—	—	—	—	100
Mo: St Louis Co	180,000	428	267	100	23	37	—	—	—	48	11	18	10	2	4	59
New York City	1,000,000	1653	875	58	4	7	110	7	13	64	4	7	32	2	4	31
New York: Rome	N/A	260	247	—	—	—	—	—	—	—	—	—	31	12	13	13
Oregon: Portland	172,674	309	171	29	9	17	69	22	40	20	6	12	37	12	22	91
Pa: Sat. Prog.	407,953	121	28	—	—	—	7	6	25	8	7	29	13	11	46	100
Pa: WPSD	N/A	447	440	—	—	—	—	—	—	59	13	13	12	3	3	16
Tenn: Nashville	85,000	147	73	6	4	8	7	5	10	5	3	7	46	31	63	88
Utah	317,332	420	83	—	—	—	—	—	—	40	10	48	37	9	44	92
Va: Fairfax Co.	134,000	342	56	13	4	23	3	1	5	23	7	41	5	2	9	78
TOTALS		4696	2642 (56.8%)	245		11.5%	254		15.3%	297		17.2%	294		22.1%	M=73.67%

Pattern 1: hearing-impaired children enrolled in an ordinary class with support from an itinerant teacher.
Pattern 2: enrolment in an ordinary class with a resource room and resource teacher in the same building.
Pattern 3: enrolment in a special class for deaf children and attendance in a hearing class for one or more academic subjects per day.
Pattern 4: enrolment in a special class and attending a class with hearing children exclusively for non-academic subjects such as physical education, art or a pre-vocational or vocational class.

* Abstracted from: Brill, R.G. (1978) *Mainstreaming the Prelingually Deaf Child.* Washington, D.C.: Gallaudet College Press, Tables A and B.

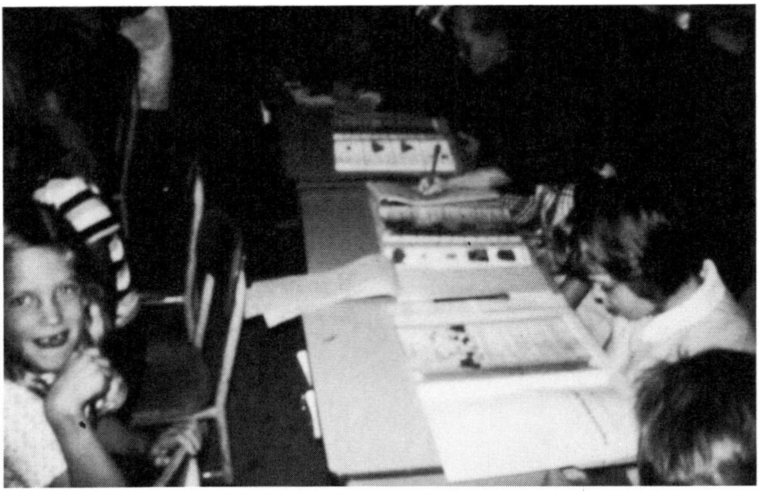
A

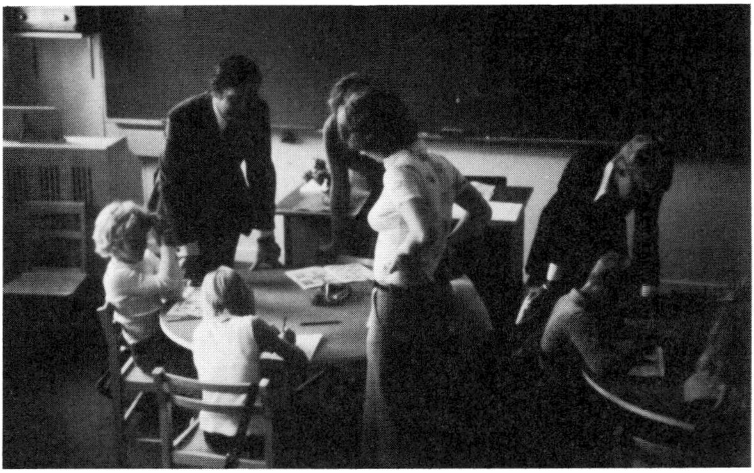
B

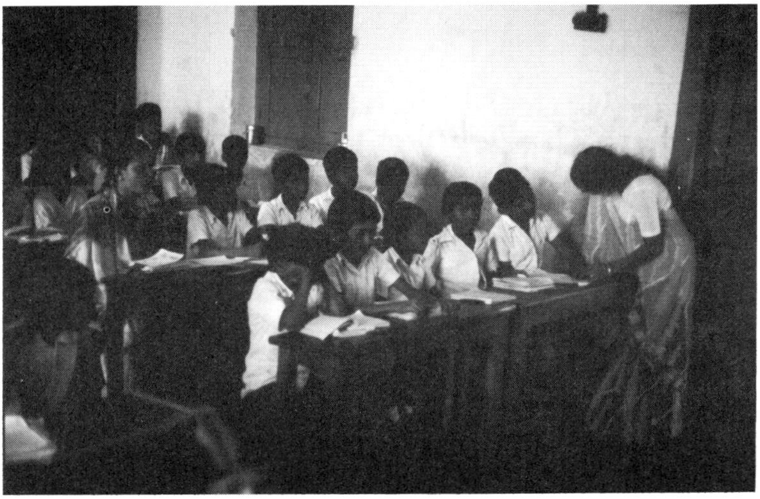
C

D

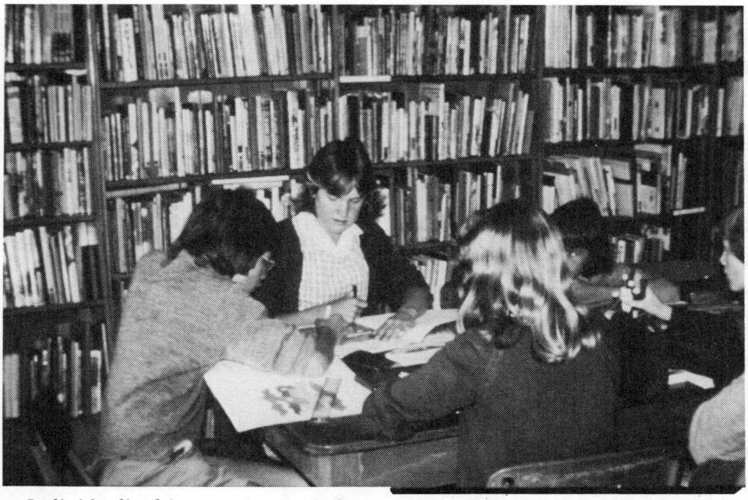

Figure 7 Individualised integration in different countries: (a) Utah, USA; (b) Linköping, Sweden; (c) Mysore, India; (d) Auckland, New Zealand.

877 mandated that every child requiring special educational treatment should have a 'core' programme. A 'core' evaluation team, including every professional who was involved with the education of a child and also the child's parents, determined the goals and the programme to be followed for each child every six months. Evaluations were by standardised tests, teacher-made tests and subjective judgements.

It was the objective in Massachusetts that every handicapped child should be integrated 'to some degree' and individual differences determined the extent to which this occurred. From Table 3 it can be seen that 88 per cent of the prelingually severely deaf children in Massachusetts in 1975–6 were integrated in one or other of Brill's four patterns. Only 8.5 per cent of these children, however, were individually integrated and assisted by itinerant teachers, while 46.3 per cent were attending special classes and attending ordinary classes only for non-academic subjects, such as art and physical education.

In all the 12 districts surveyed by Dr Brill, 4696 children were recorded as hearing-impaired and, of these, 2642 were severely or profoundly hearing-impaired (average pure tone losses in the better ear of 70 dB or greater). Of these 2642 children, 1090 (41.3 per cent) were attending ordinary schools. Only 245 or 23 per cent of these 1090 severely deaf children appeared to be individually integrated in their local ordinary schools and served by itinerant teachers of the deaf. The remaining 77 per cent attended ordinary schools with resource classes or special unit classes.

There were, however, large variations in percentages of children individually integrated in local schools within the 12 districts (Table 3). In St Louis County (Missouri), for example, 37 per cent of the severely or profoundly deaf children were individually integrated in their local schools, and in Fairfax County (Virginia) and Minnesota Special District, 23 per cent. In four other districts, no severely deaf children were individually integrated, and the overall percentage for all of the 12 districts was 11.5 per cent. It should be remembered that these regions were selected because they were 12 of the 15 most 'main-streamed' areas in the United States in 1975–6.

One of the most interesting of these 12 US programmes was that in St Louis County, Missouri, and fortunately this was described in detail by Dr V.V. Yater in 1977.[236] The parents of 40 main-streamed children attending 29 schools in 14 school districts responded to a questionnaire sent by Dr Yater to 72 homes. All of these 40 children had attended schools or classes for hearing-impaired children prior to their being integrated. Twelve had hearing losses of 100 dB or greater and nine had losses of between 90 and 100 dB, and all 40 children received regular assistance from hearing-aid clinicians while in the ordinary schools. Unfortunately, no breakdown of time spent individually with each child was given.

The reports of nearly all parents, class teachers and audiologists were, overall, very positive indeed. Of the 21 most deaf children, 14 became deaf at birth, two between the ages of one and two, three between two and three, and one each between three and four and four and five years.

The IQs of the whole group of 40 children were basically within the normal range (WISC and Wechsler Pre-school Primary Scale of Intelligence) although nine of them were in the superior range of intelligence on the performance scale and 'a few students had superior full-scale scores'. Yater commented (p. 52) that 'the single most important variable in helping to decide which child should be main-streamed was that of *intellectual capability*.'

Parents of students who had been main-streamed for a longer period, and the students themselves, felt that both social development and academic attainment improved after an initial period of adjustment to the new school environment. The question may be asked: 'Should most of these 40 children have been segregated in the first place?' One must consider whether they might not have been better placed at the outset in their local ordinary schools. The 'integration readiness' to which Yater and others have referred appears to this writer to depend more on the amount of support available once the child is in the ordinary school, than on a child's language development or even social adjustment prior to entry (*see* chapters 5, 6, 8 and 9).

Yater considered four 'readiness factors' – the child, the school, support professionals and the parents – and useful suggestions were made in considering these (pp. 52–9). She suggested that these were flexible and could be altered if one or more of them appeared negative. Even so, she felt that a child incapable of taking the verbal portion of the WISC was not suitable for consideration and that achievement tests could be another pre-placement step towards integration.

Useful studies of integration at the tertiary level have been conducted by staff of the Rochester National Technical Institute for the Deaf in New York State. R. Riffer, for example, studied student attitudes and social patterns existing between deaf and normally hearing students attending this large technical institute after it began admitting severely deaf students in 1969.[188] (By December 1978, 850 hearing-impaired students had been admitted and the total full-time enrolment of both deaf and normally hearing students was 6258.[188])

Close friendships between deaf and normally hearing students were more common when the deaf student had intelligible speech and after the normally hearing students had spent time with resident adviser/student interpreters. Riffer concluded:

> While integration to an extent has been achieved for a greater portion of deaf students through separate housing, it has been on the deaf students' terms with the small number of hearing students entering the sub-culture of the deaf rather than the deaf students moving into the larger hearing students' culture.

It had not been possible to conduct a study of the reciprocity of feelings of friendship from hearing to deaf student although this would have been most useful.

Sharing classes with normally hearing students did not seem in itself to lead to more friendships with hearing students. Riffer inferred that what occurred outside the classroom was more important than interaction within it for leading to meaningful social interaction between deaf and hearing students. It is emphasised here, however, that when deaf students attend ordinary classes individually, much more interaction occurs.[102] (*See* the Sheffield, Derby and London further education reports in chapter 8, page 112 *et seq.*)

It is possible that, in the 53 other college/career programmes for deaf students which have recently been established in the United States,[183] opportunities for individual attendance in classes will have shown a more positive degree of integration and the establishment of a larger number of warm relationships. In fact, 31 of the 137 courses in 1974 and 72 of the 275 courses taken by deaf students in the United States in 1978 were each followed by one student only. Some other courses, for example, fashion, design, library science, child care, journalism, electrical engineering, and dental technology, were followed by two or three students, but in two or three different colleges. In these 90 or so cases, it is expected that much greater social integration would have occurred.

Support services offered to the hearing-impaired students in all the above programmes included special classes for deaf students; signing or oral interpreters in ordinary classes; tutoring; note-taking; vocational development and placement courses; personal counselling; social/cultural services; speech and hearing services; and manual communication training for deaf students. Parsons, in 1979, observed that parents of deaf students in some 'Total Communication'[117] programmes were extremely concerned that their children had not developed intelligible speech, or that their speech had deteriorated. In part, Parsons felt* that this accounted for the current enthusiasm for speech programmes in the United States.[31,141]

* Personal communication from M.B. Parsons following his Alexander G. Bell Association International Lecturer's tour of the United States.

D.B. Gjerdingen has listed over 100 colleges and universities where ex-students of the Central Institute for the Deaf (CID) in St Louis, Missouri, have completed university degrees.[102] He indicated that these bright deaf students do not have to restrict themselves to 'special colleges for the deaf, such as Gallaudet College and the National Technical Institute for the Deaf, or colleges where a special programme exists for accommodating the curriculum and instruction procedures, such as that of California State University at Northbridge'. It was important, he went on, for deaf students to be aware 'that broader opportunities are also possible – at least for some deaf students'.

Most of the institutions of higher learning selected by these CID students 'did not have special provisions for helping deaf students', and they ranged from small schools and colleges to giant multi-universities like those of Michigan and Southern California. 'The choices our deaf alumni have made are as varied and unrestricted as those of students with normal hearing.'

Although no formal educational support programme existed in these colleges, it is unlikely that *no* assistance was offered them and, doubtless, parents and lecturers would have arranged individual coaching sessions, additional printed handouts and so on, as have been found useful in other examples mentioned in chapter 8. The ways in which the other students, the staff and parents *had* assisted these deaf students would make another excellent research study.

New Zealand

A most helpful, though disturbing, study was carried out by M. Vandenberg of 77 children who wore hearing aids and attended 58 ordinary schools in and around Wellington, New Zealand, in 1970.[227] Data was collected by means of two questionnaires. The one for teachers, taking 30–40 minutes to complete, sought information on each child's communication ability, emotional adjustment and classroom behaviour; whether additional help should be provided, and if so, what form it should take; and, finally, details of any training the teacher had had for assisting a hearing-impaired child. The children's questionnaire (a structured interview) took an average of 20 minutes to administer. Vandenberg commented that the time taken to administer the questionnaire often depended on the loquaciousness of the child. 'A number of the children so obviously enjoyed the one-to-one situation and the experience of being able to do successfully what was asked of them, that they tended to give more expansive answers than were called for.'

Reading and arithmetic results were both depressed by comparison with normally hearing children of the same age and intelligence. Hearing aids were not worn by the least deaf 25 per cent of the group and were rarely worn by a further 20 per cent.

There was an almost total lack of class teacher preparation for assisting a hearing-impaired child. One of the conclusions was that non-specialist teachers (after expert advice) should offer many of these children 'individualised help, preferably on a daily basis until the need for such help was no longer required'. It seemed to Mrs Vandenberg that such help would be of most benefit to the younger children who were in the process of acquiring language and academic skills and had not by then had too many unrewarding and inhibiting experiences of failure. Specialist teachers visited the less deaf children infrequently and useful notes on ways of helping these children were not automatically passed on from one class teacher to another at the end of each year.

One-fifth of the children were felt by their teachers to be much quieter and less communicative than their classmates. Twenty-one of the 77 children said that they had no close friends at home, and five had no close friends at school. The following disturbing comments were made when four of the children were interviewed:

1 I play with no one in the playground. Mostly walk around, that's all. I'm thinking of getting a tape recorder that will tell me what the teacher will do next day and the teacher will say, 'You've done everything I told you to do.' I lunch with no one at school. I try and make myself sit by myself and have a bit of peace and that's all I want at home. At home I like best to be with my toys as they don't talk to me unless I ask them to.
2 I have no best friend. I have nobody to play with at school. I like everybody but they don't like me. I just play by myself in the playground. I don't know what to do. Just sit at home, knit a scarf or something, tidy up the house one or two days a year.
3 I haven't any friends. No one plays with me. I just sit around and walk. That's why I like going home for lunch. Whenever I can, I make excuses to go home.
4 What I like least about school is the kids not letting me play games and all that – because I don't want to be lonely. I just hang around the school looking at something.

A number of Vandenberg's and James and James's findings (like those of the Department of Education and Science report of 1963[79] and H.L. Owrid and P. Hamilton in 1972[170]) give cause for real concern, and reflect the need for considerable and *continuing* care and effort when handicapped children are being educated in ordinary classrooms.

These results should, however, be compared with studies such as those in New Zealand in 1976 reported in chapter 6 – and in other studies in this chapter and in chapter 5. Here, much more severely handicapped children *have* made worthwhile home and school friendships and have achieved more satisfactory school attainments. The importance of additional training courses for ordinary school teachers and of regular assistance to these children by additional teachers and helpers, is clearly indicated – not only with academic work but also in social situations. Social workers and home assistants (chapter 9), by working in close collaboration with teachers and parents, are also making an increasingly positive contribution towards making schooling both worthwhile and pleasant.

Argentina

A very interesting programme has operated in Argentina since 1955.[10] Dr Jose Bello, an otologist and lecturer in otolaryngology at the University of Buenos Aires, began a clinic – the Centro de Rehabilitacion Diana – having been influenced in 1955 by W.G. Hardy of John Hopkins Hospital, Baltimore, and Mrs Spencer Tracy, Director of the John Tracy Clinic in Los Angeles. In 1955, Hardy had insisted that 99.99 per cent of 'deaf' children had remnants of useful hearing and Mrs Tracy taught Dr Bello that a child who was born deaf should receive his early education from his mother. Bello considered that this should begin from the second month of the child's life – with babbling and taking advantage of other environmental sounds.

Basing their approach largely on that of the John Tracy Clinic, by 1974 Bello and his colleagues had come to a number of conclusions, such as:

(1) The education of the mother (and father) in *all* aspects relating to the education of their child was essential. Not only the specialised aspects of teaching – for example, the use and maintenance of hearing aids, the technicalities of articulation and the organisation of language – but also the role that home plays in the development of an affectionate and secure personality. 'Mother and home are the mainstays in the rehabilitation scheme.'
(2) Education should be begun as soon as the diagnosis of deafness was made, because 'the capacity to learn and adapt is always greater in the very young'.
(3) Contact with other deaf children should be avoided. This remarkable and, I believe, unique statement was implemented with such fidelity that appointments at the audiology clinic were spaced so that two deaf children would never meet.
(4) For school-aged children, special education should be given *individually* whenever possible, and teaching schemes which were divided into grades should be avoided.

It is unfortunate that Bello did not provide details of hearing losses, aetiologies, ages of onset of deafness, assessments of intelligence, nor details of home backgrounds. However, the programme, which has run for 25 years, seems worthy of much closer study.

5

Research in London 1971–7 and a survey in Norfolk

Studies in London

As a result of observations made in England and New Zealand and in the Rocklands County programme near New York (September 1970), where several severely deaf children were attending ordinary school classes individually for large portions of each school day, it was decided to mount an investigation into the question of individualised integration.

A pilot study initiated by the writer in six south London schools in 1971 indicated that support teachers for individually integrated, hearing-impaired children who worked in the classrooms would be warmly welcomed by ordinary school teachers, as well as by the children and their parents. Six students of special education at Avery Hill College of Education carried out this study and found the work full of interest (Fig. 8). At the conclusion of the six-week study, four of the hearing-impaired children commented that they had had to work harder, but that they had enjoyed school more while the support teacher had been at their school.

In 1972, the chief education officer in the north London borough of Haringey agreed that a longitudinal study could be undertaken by the University of London Institute of Education in collaboration with the authority's officer for special education and the head teacher of the school for deaf children.[52] The speech production[62,203] and reading attainments[68,108] of all the testable children in the Haringey deaf school and units were measured in April and June 1972, and again between May and July 1973 (*see* chapter 10).

Six children (mean age 10.3 years; mean hearing loss 76.7 decibels [dB]) from the junior school unit were placed in their local ordinary schools in May 1973; seven other children who remained in the unit were selected as controls (Table 4, page 69). The academic ability of both the experimental group and the control group was rated as average by their teachers, but the educational

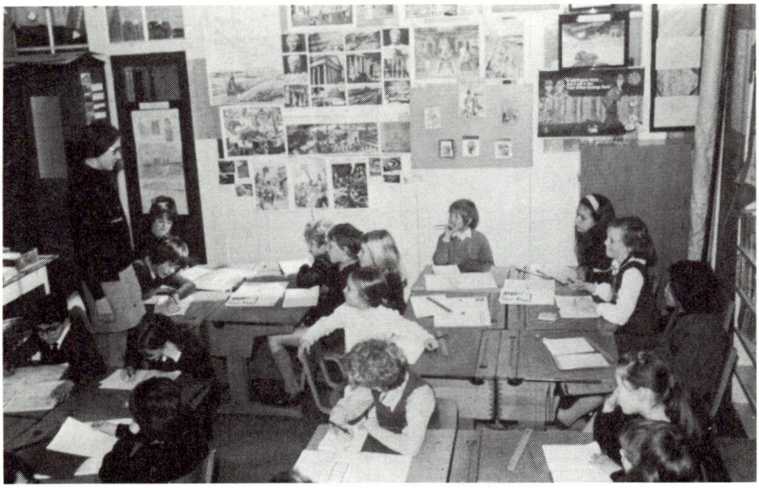

A

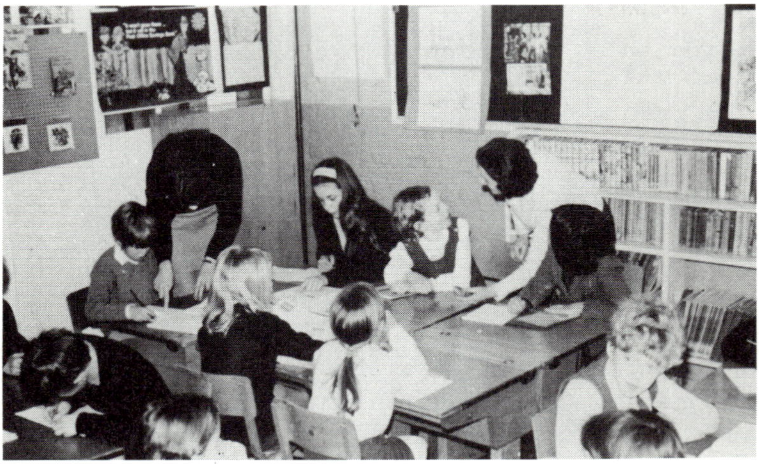

B

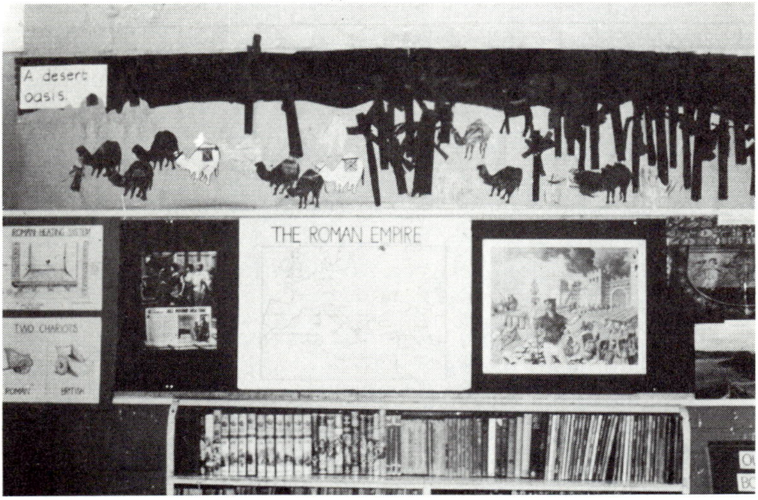

C

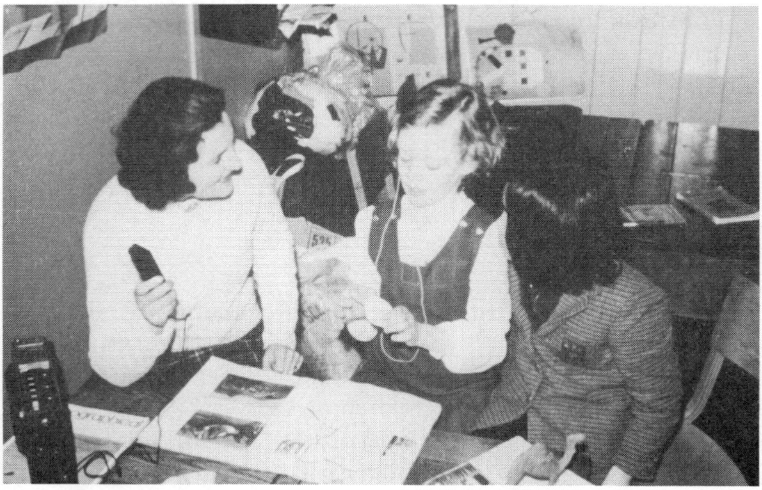
D

Figure 8 A pilot study of support teaching for individually integrated children, conducted in south London in 1971.
(a) The class teacher uses a microphone incorporating a radio transmitter for the hearing impaired child. (b) The class teacher and support teacher work together. (c) The class have studied 'People who live in the desert' for four weeks and have made a wall picture (above). (d) The support teacher revises an oral lesson with a hearing-impaired child and a normally hearing child needing remedial help.

potential of the homes of all but one of the experimental group was considered to be below average. (*See* Appendix 3, pp. 170–3.)

The experiment was begun after careful preparation, and full discussions were held with Mr W.H. Snowdon, Her Majesty's Inspector of Special Schools (who had begun his career as a teacher of deaf children). Local inspectors and advisers were also consulted regarding the suitability of schools in this rather poor area of north London. Head teachers recommended class teachers in their schools whom they considered to be both competent and interested. The head teachers and this writer then approached these teachers to explain how it was hoped the programme would function, and to ask them if they would consider becoming involved in the scheme after they had been to see the child to be integrated and had had a discussion with his or her teacher of the deaf in the unit. The parents of the six experimental children were invited to the school for the deaf one evening when the head teacher spoke to them about the project, explaining how a teacher of the deaf and three other teachers were to be employed to help the class teachers in helping their children.

Slides were shown of the earlier work in south London mentioned above. It was emphasised to the parents that, if the deaf children were unhappy with this new scheme, or the ordinary schools were dissatisfied for some reason, the experiment would be discontinued. Places were to be kept for all six children in the unit classes they had left, so that any return would not be difficult. All parents seemed reassured by this and all agreed that their child should be placed in his or her local ordinary school.

In addition to their individual hearing aids, radio transmitter hearing aids were also purchased for four of the six children to help overcome the poor acoustic conditions in the ordinary school classrooms. Three small slide projectors and three language masters were purchased, particularly to help in the micro-teaching unit (*see* Fig. 8). These were shared between the six children.

The preliminary stage

Because the project was experimental and a large proportion of children in the schools (and the research group) came from immigrant families, support in this initial stage was particularly generous. One teacher of the deaf and three support teachers assisted these six children on transfer.

It was recognised that the class teacher of normally hearing children could not spare a great deal of time to teach the hearing-impaired child. It was hoped, however, that he or she would be able to assist in the following ways:

* ★ Discuss – with the teacher of deaf children and the assistant (support) teacher – the syllabus to be attempted with the normally hearing class, the individual programme designed by the teacher of the deaf, and the results of the previous day's programme. This would enable the teacher of the deaf to plan complementary programmes to back up what the deaf child missed in ordinary lessons.
* ★ Briefly supervise the individual language, reading and auditory training exercises provided by the teacher of the deaf.
* ★ Bring the hearing-impaired children into conversations and discussion wherever possible.
* ★ Encourage the normally hearing children to bring the deaf child into their conversations and group discussions.

It was anticipated that the teacher of deaf children would:

* ★ Give individual speech and language teaching to the deaf child for up to 45 minutes every day.
* ★ Evaluate the previous day's programmes attempted by the deaf child and construct new ones each day.
* ★ Liaise as closely as possible with the class teacher (and head teacher) on all aspects of the deaf child's educational and social development.
* ★ Guide and encourage the half-time assistant (support) teachers each day.
* ★ Administer periodical audiological, educational and social adjustment tests to the children.
* ★ Visit the homes of the deaf children regularly with the support teacher to hear their problems and give appropriate guidance, and
* ★ Generally take responsibility for the deaf child's success or otherwise in the programme.

The three assistant/support teachers who, in the south London pilot study, had been found to be of very great importance, were to spend half of each day with each deaf child. They would be able to assist in a variety of ways which would include the following:

* ★ Interpret information such as school or class announcements to help ensure that the deaf child understood what was going on in school.
* ★ Spend up to 45 minutes in school with each child in the study, discussing home news and current events, hearing reading, and giving assistance with other aspects of school work recommended by the class teacher or teacher of the deaf or requested by the child.
* ★ Conduct a further session of approximately 30 minutes of micro-teaching unit work. Two or three of the children from the class were to join the research child in reading, mathematics or some other topic which the class teacher felt would be of benefit to them all.
* ★ Set up, under the general guidance and supervision of the teacher of the deaf, apparatus for individual programmes which could be supervised by the class teacher in reading, language and auditory training, using film strips, slides, language master, tape recorder and 8 mm cine-loop films for lipreading practice.
* ★ By example and precept, encourage the normally hearing children to bring the handicapped child into group conversations and activities and accept him/her casually but warmly.
* ★ Report daily, either verbally or in writing, to the itinerant teacher of the deaf.
* ★ Report in very considerable detail, to parents the significant events of each school day.
* ★ Keep a daily diary of events which is submitted by the teacher of the deaf each week to the head teacher of the school for deaf children and to the university research unit (*see below*).

The parents were now felt to be in a position to receive an unprecedented amount of information about their child's progress at school. They were encouraged to:

* ★ Work as conscientiously as possible through the home/school book each evening and discuss with their children significant happenings reported there, not only in brief evening sessions, but also - and perhaps more importantly - on subsequent incidental occasions, as the material arose in real life.
* ★ Report to the teacher of the deaf and the support teacher significant happenings in the home, such as 'My husband brought home a new electric drill last night. He will make John and Terry some bunk beds,' or 'Terry fell off his bike last night. He skinned his knee but he didn't cry,' or 'Terry says "London" very clearly. Can you please ask him to say it for you?'
* ★ Make occasional school visits as well as expect the home visits by the teacher of the deaf and the support teachers once each term.

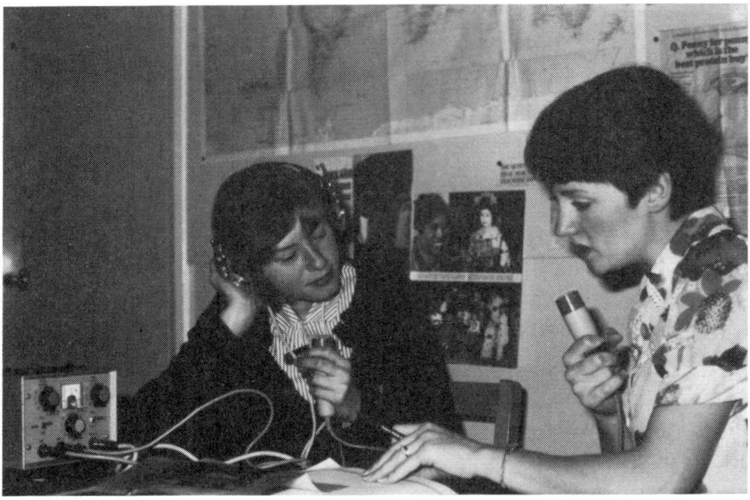

A

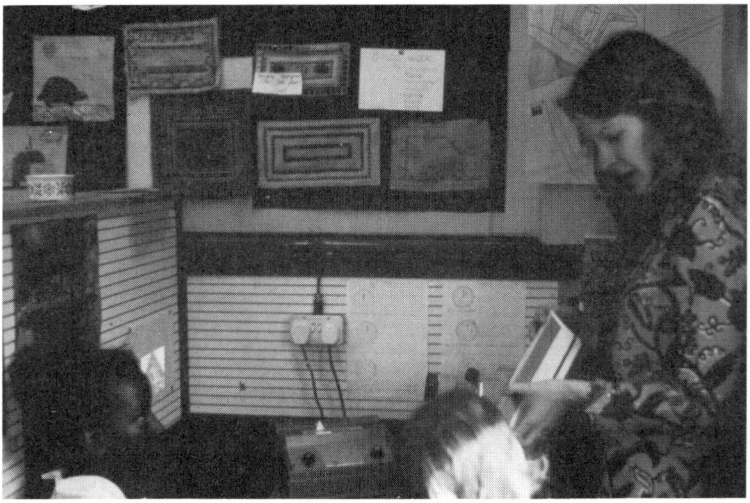

B

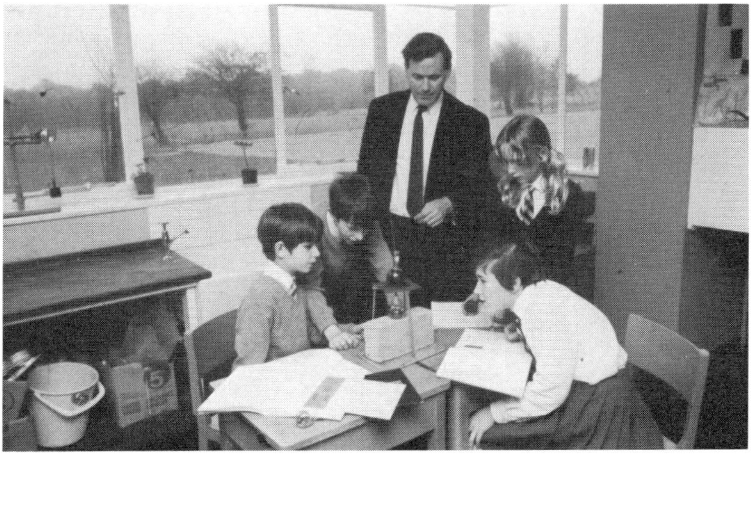

C

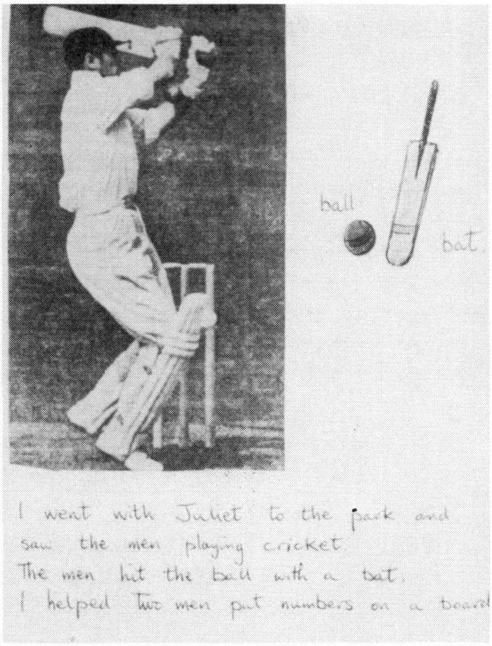

D

Figure 9 Assistance from an itinerant teacher of the deaf, support teacher and class teacher, and the parents' family diary.
(a) Daily speech teaching. (b) A support teacher helps a deaf child and a backward reader to use a Language Master. (c) A class teacher aids three normally hearing children and one deaf child. (Experiments are often introduced and followed up by the teacher of the deaf or the support teacher.) (d) A daily family diary – one of the best aids to reading that parents can provide.

Supervision and assessments

Regular meetings with the itinerant teacher of the deaf and the support teachers were held with the head teacher at the deaf school. (This writer also devoted at least one full day each week to the project.)

In addition to the reading and speech measurements noted above, regular observations of, and interviews with, teachers, parents and children were conducted – both hearing-impaired and normally hearing. By August 1973 it was possible to report the following:

> In May this year, the six children from the Risley Avenue hearing-impaired unit began attending their local junior schools with additional support. Despite some points which have given concern, the experiment to date shows distinct promise.
>
> *Parents:* Visits to homes by the teacher of the deaf and the support teachers have created an interest where, in some cases, little seemed to exist previously. Results of a questionnaire given to the parents of the six research children towards the end of the term indicated their general satisfaction with the way the experiment was running.
>
> *Attainment tests:* Tests of reading and speech production were administered in April 1972, and in May 1973 [Appendix 3]. The tests were repeated in July 1973, but with such a small sample and such a short period of time, no conclusive differences in results were obtained. In the Hamp word

recognition test, for example, an average improvement of 0.31 of one year was obtained in nine weeks compared with 0.20 of one year in the whole of the previous year in the hearing-impaired unit. The difference was not statistically significant, however.

No significant difference was found in the children's articulation of speech phonemes although slight improvements in scores were recorded.

By normally hearing children's standards, the results suggested quite severe educational retardation, five of the six children rating as 'backward' in reading (i.e. reading ages more than two years below their chronological ages), and speech grossly defective in one case and seriously affected in two others. Such results are not uncommon with hearing-impaired children, although it is hoped that some such strategy as the experimental provision might eventually bring their attainments up significantly.

Support teachers made a more positive assessment of the children's progress than was shown by the tests. Two children were felt to have made 'exceptional' and three 'good' progress in speech production; two were felt to have made 'good' progress in reading and four 'satisfactory' progress. No child was rated as having made 'little' or 'no' progress in speech, language or reading.

Social adjustment: During this term, it was interesting to observe that parents in the case of three children, and teachers in the case of all six, noted welcome developments in social adjustment and behaviour. One boy was felt to be using his voice more in conversation and was signing and gesturing much less. Another boy began to discuss things with his parents in a way that was quite foreign to him previously. A third was working much harder with his homework and had shown a welcome growth in responsibility to his parents and other members of the family. A nine-year-old girl who was previously staying out late at night and arriving late for school, was, by the end of the term, going to bed by 8.30 or 9.00 p.m. and was rarely late for school. One of the girls who, at the outset, tried too hard to make friends and was somewhat disappointed, became accepted quite warmly by a number of the normally hearing children.

Comments by support and class teachers regarding the children were, on the whole, very favourable. All felt that the six children had been at least 'reasonably happy' both in and out of school. Support teachers felt that only one child had not made a best friend in the normally hearing class; however, three of the class teachers believed that three of the children had not made a best friend during the ten-week period in the ordinary school. Eight of the twelve ratings indicated that casual friendships had formed with *most* members of the class, and three others that such friendships had been observed with *a number* of the other children.

From September 1973 to April 1974 it is proposed to continue the overall teaching and assessment programme along the lines suggested in the notes above. It is hoped that this writer can:

(a) encourage even closer planning of work between support and class teachers.
(b) visit all six homes to learn more about their difficulties and to guide and encourage the parents to participate more fully in the education of their children.
(c) spend half-days with support teachers every three weeks, rather than one-sixth of a day with them each week, specifically to study and assist the collaboration with class teachers, and to experiment further in using language masters, cine-loop projectors, etc.
(d) spend more time with the teacher of the deaf to ascertain more clearly how such a teacher's time might best be spent.
(e) retest all the school for the deaf and the unit children aged between six and 13 years to continue the longitudinal study which was begun in 1972 and to obtain sufficient cases as control groups and for any expansion of the project.

When one of the three support teachers had to be absent for ten days in September 1973, it was possible for this writer to substitute for her on eight of those days and to make the following report:

> The overall impression gained was of a most attractive teaching post with innumerable opportunities for presenting stimulating language, reading and speech to the two children involved. (Both girls were nine years old; Jacqueline had a hearing loss of 80 decibels and Alexandra 90 decibels.) My functions as a support teacher involved the following:
>
> *Revision* of oral material presented by the class teacher, the head teachers at assemblies and during music sessions, other teachers and children. Much of this material was first written in the childrens' home/school exercise books which I found I used very frequently.
> *Language:* As well as observing language work conducted by the class teacher, it was necessary to introduce other materials from the Language Topics, Sections I, II and III, which could meet the colloquial language needs of these children more nearly.[56]
> *News:* Each morning we had a daily news session. Each child told of interesting happenings at home and these were put into conversational language forms.[228] The most interesting were written for them in their home/school books, using direct speech whenever possible. In addition, a few items of my home news were given, photographs of my children shown and so on, and both girls seemed to appreciate this. Items from the newspaper were sometimes discussed and wall maps and atlases were consulted to identify the locations of the various happenings. (The child would normally bring a jotter pad and pencil to the news session.)
> *Reading:* Useful opportunities exist for providing the children with daily reading materials – experience reading, reading exercises and reading from set books. I am not happy, however, about the books which I used and hope to see a variety of readers available to the children and a record kept

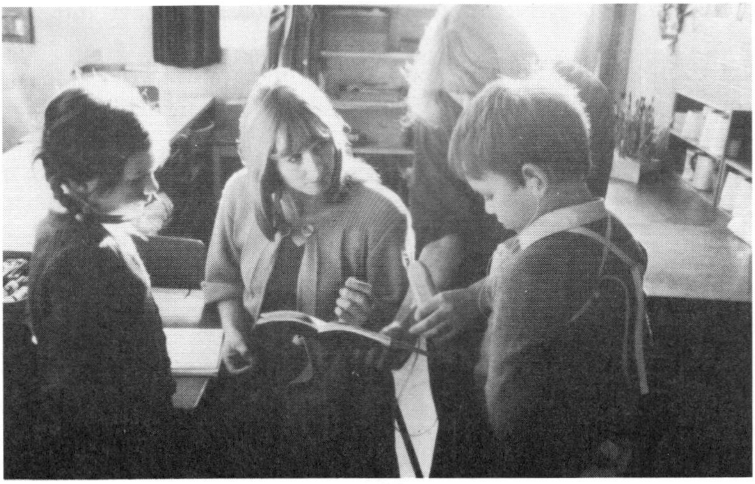

A

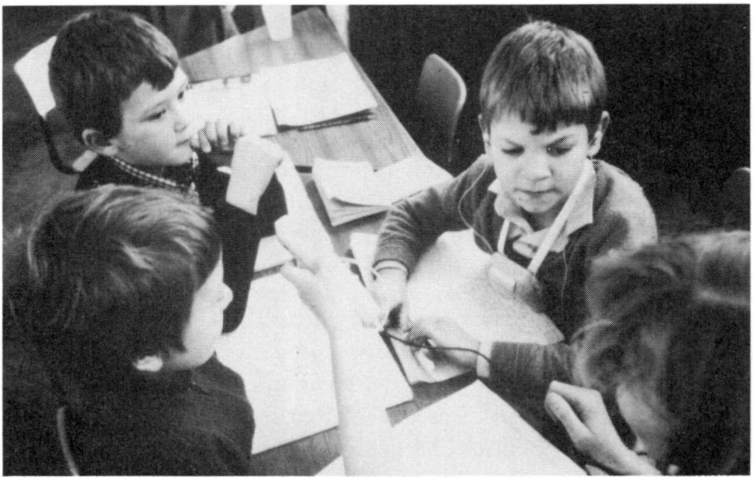

B

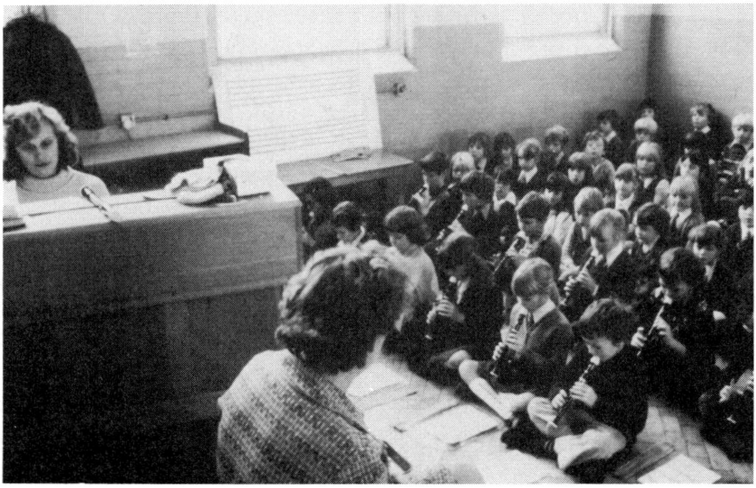

C

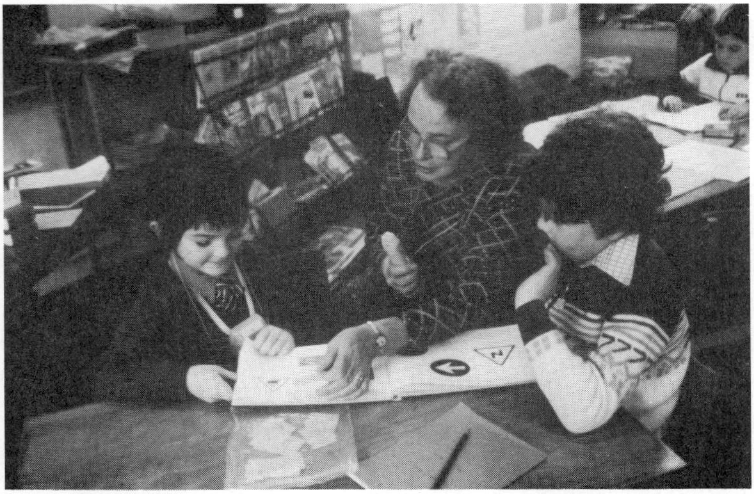

D

Figure 10 Team teaching: assistance from class teachers, head teacher, welfare assistant, classmates and teacher of the deaf in a Portsmouth school, 1980.
(a) Specialist and class teacher discuss a reading difficulty. A normally hearing child also learns about the problems of deafness.
(b) The teacher of the deaf passes the microphone to one of the normally hearing children during a language lesson.
(c) The head teacher conducts a recorder lesson. The 100 dB deaf boy is in the second row. A welfare assistant plays the piano accompaniment.
(d) A class teacher helps a profoundly deaf boy to read while his friend and reading partner observes.

of the interest shown in the various titles. (Daily oral reading is felt to be of critical importance to these children.)[103] Two simple dictionaries have been ordered for each of the children to use frequently at home as well as at school.

Apparatus: The language master was carried daily between the two schools, and proved to be of interest to the research children and the normally hearing boys and girls as well [Fig. 10]. I hope that we can extend the uses of the instrument over the next few weeks, using cards prepared by teachers but also trade materials, and question and answer cards of some mathematics as well as language work. The radio transmitter hearing aids functioned fairly well but were not used as frequently as they should have been. They should certainly be used at all assemblies and all other occasions in the hall and rather more than I used them in the classroom. When a class teacher is conducting a class lesson, story-telling, etc., she should be asked to wear the radio transmitter.

Mathematics: The children were both asked to work on the 24-hour clock but neither had much idea about this, and there were not sufficient exercises in the *Beta Mathematics Book 3* to give them sufficient practice. We should look more closely at a mathematics scheme for these children.

Speech: Excellent situations existed for teaching speech relevant to each child's needs. Work covered was written in the child's home/school books for practice in everyday situations at home. Assistant teachers should daily inform the teacher of the deaf of words and phrases which have been said particularly well or which need improving.

Parents: Perhaps the most disturbing aspect of this eight-day exercise was the lack of response achieved from the parents. It is clear that neither of the homes appreciate yet what is required if they are to make the most of their unique educational opportunities. A meeting of all parents will be arranged within the next three weeks.

Integration: One has to think of situations for the handicapped and unhandicapped children to mix happily during the preparation of each day's work. A Lotto game using simple arithmetic exercises proved successful, as did the language master work mentioned above and activities such as pitching a small tent in the park beside the school. Genuine friendships have developed well between the research children and several of the normally hearing ones.

By July 1974 it was possible to report as follows:

Results to date are most encouraging: none of the six children wishes to return to the hearing-impaired unit; the parents of all six children are enthusiastic that the experiment should continue; the head teachers of the junior schools are very much in favour of such provision and would be pleased to admit other hearing-handicapped children on a similar basis; the class teachers and assistant teachers (despite fairly frequent visits in the last term by interested teachers and doctors) have coped well and both groups of teachers appear to have found the work interesting and worthwhile. The teacher of the deaf appointed to the experiment in May 1973 is now most enthusiastic about the possibilities of this method of teaching hearing impaired children.

Assessments: It has been shown that reading vocabulary ages[108] have in all cases accelerated (in four cases markedly) this year compared with the progress these children achieved in the hearing-impaired unit last year – overall mean = 1.03 years progress, as opposed to only 0.20 of one year [Table 4, Fig. 9]. Progress achieved on the same test by 15 children who remained in the partially hearing unit this year was 0.113 of one year.

Gains in speech articulation[62] were recorded in the experimental situation in all cases, and parents reported that five out of the six children were speaking 'a little more clearly' and talking 'much more' at home than when they attended the unit for hearing-impaired children; the sixth child was said to be speaking 'a little more clearly' and 'a little more'.

Results from Rutter (Parent and Teacher Social Adjustment Schedules)[195] and weekly observations of teachers indicated that, in five cases, the children had improved significantly in social adjustment during the course of the individual integration experiment. The capacity of the six children to make and retain friendships was observed closely throughout the year. All six children, according to the assistant teachers, had made at

Table 4 Reading vocabulary ages and speech articulation scores in Experimental Group 1 and controls, 1972–7

	Reading age (years) (Hamp test)						Consonant articulation (Dale)				Mean rate of utterance (Spencer)	
	April 1972*	May 1973*	May 1974	June 1975	June 1976	June 1977	April 1972	May 1973	June 1976	June 1977	June 1976	June 1977
Experimental group I (5)† Hearing loss 79.0 ± 11.6 dB	7.7 ± 0.3 (7.4–8.0)	7.9 ± 0.6 (7.3–8.5)	8.6 ± 0.7 (7.8–9.0)	9.1 ± 0.9 (8.0–9.4)	9.4 ± 0.9 (8.3–10.3)‡	10.3 ± 0.9 (9.2–11.4)‡	11.8 ± 4.7	13.8 ± 5.7	20.0 ± 2.1	20.0 ± 2.9	5.3 ± 1.5	4.5 ± 0.8
Controls Group 1 (from units) (7) Hearing loss	7.2 ± 0.3 (6.8–7.6	7.5 ± 0.4 (7.1–7.9	7.5 ± 0.4 (7.3–8.1)	7.5 ± 0.4 (7.3–8.5)	8.0 0.5 (7.5–8.5)	8.4 ± 0.6 (7.8–9.0)	10.0 ± 2.8	11.6 ± 3.6	18.4 ± 3.3	15.9 ± 2.6	5.1 ± 1.0	5.0 ± 1.0
From school for deaf (9) Hearing loss 103 ± 6.3 dB	6.6 ± 1.3	7.3 ± 1.4	7.6 ± 1.3	7.6 ± 0.6	8.0 ± 0.9	8.2 ± 1.0	4.3 ± 7.1	4.8 ± 4.8	10.0 ± 9.2	12.3 ± 8.6	6.3 ± 2.9	5.7 ± 1.5

* Assessments made before individual integration. Results are mean ± S.D. (range).
† Results from only those of the group who remained in the study from 1972–77.
‡ Results depressed because the Hamp test has a maximum of 11 years. Results with Daniels and Diack's graded test of reading experience in 1 child in 1976 (11.4 years) and 2 children in 1977 (12.9 years and 11.1 years) are not included in the table.

From *The Lancet*, 21 October 1978, by kind permission.

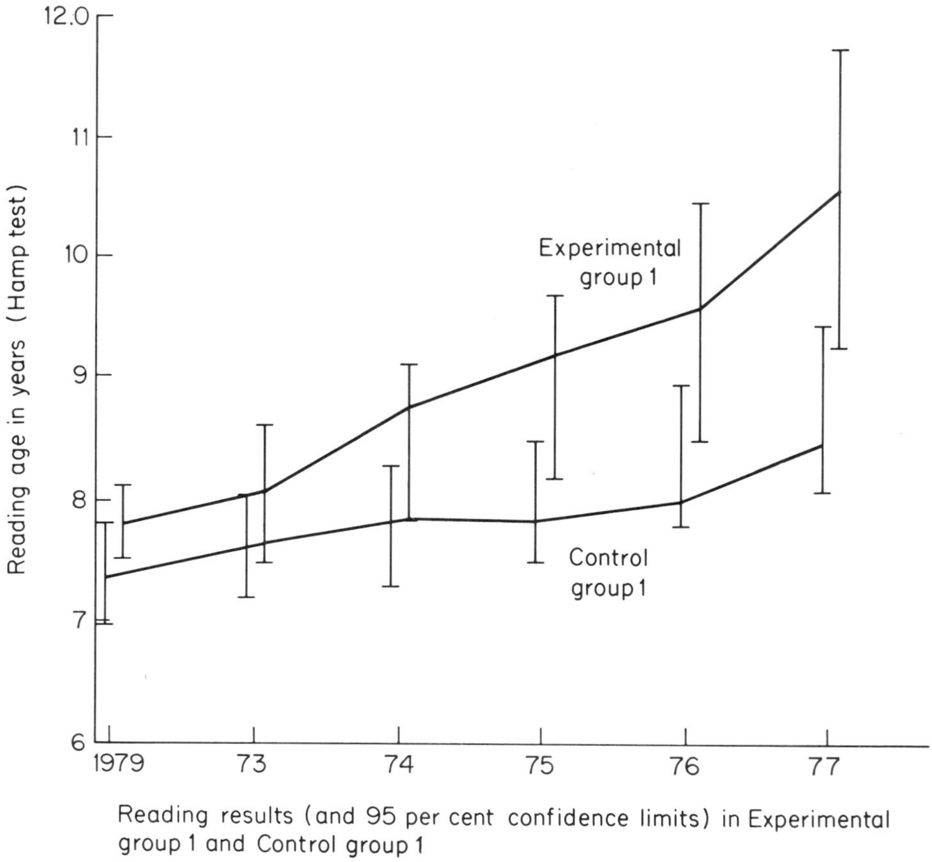

Figure 11 Reading results (and 95 per cent confidence limits) in Experimental Group 1 and Control Group 1, from the north London study, 1972–7.

least one close friend in each class (in two cases, friendships changed twice and three times respectively during the course of the year). All the children had made a large number of casual friendships.

Cost: The cost of this scheme at the present time (approximately £1300 per child) is too high. There are, however, modifications which can significantly reduce this. By including in the group of children a proportion who are not so seriously handicapped (i.e., too handicapped to cope alone in an ordinary school, but requiring only, say, one session each week from a teacher of the deaf and two from an assistant teacher) it will be possible to increase the overall number to perhaps 12 children – thus almost halving the present cost and bringing it into line with the cost of unit and day school for deaf children (£730 per annum in Haringey in 1973, *see also* Table 10, p. 138).

> *Development:* The five eldest children were enrolled in the local secondary schools of their parents' choice in September. The headmaster of the Blanche Nevile School for Deaf Children (who is involved in this research in a supervisory capacity) and I [the present writer] have visited the four secondary schools regularly and have been most encouraged by the response of the children and teachers and the opportunities which seem to be available there. The sixth child, who is a year younger than the rest, will go on to his local secondary school this September.
>
> *Need to extend the research:* Due to the small numbers so far involved, only tentative conclusions may be drawn from the research to date. There is thus an urgent need, following this encouraging beginning, to make a wider and deeper investigation involving a greater variety of children of differing ages and degrees of deafness and coming from different home conditions. If the overall findings are similarly successful, then highly significant changes in our present practice could be recommended with confidence.

Eight children were subsequently added to the experimental group, five during 1975–6 (Table 5) and three during 1976–7. Ages of these two additional groups ranged from 7.5 to 12.3 years and 6.0 to 12.8 years respectively, and hearing losses for each of the groups were 100, 100, 85 and 35 dB, and 110, 105 and 65 dB. Four of the eight subjects had been attending the school for deaf children. Teachers' estimates of academic ability were from B+ to C− (mean C). The mean home rating of these eight children was again only D (on an A–E scale where A = very helpful educationally).

By 1976 two full-time teachers of the deaf and four support teachers were engaged to give special assistance to the above 13 children.

Table 5 Reading vocabulary ages and speech articulation in Experimental Group 2 and controls, 1972–7

	Reading age		Consonant articulation		Rate of utterance	
Group	June 1976	June 1977	June 1976	June 1977	June 1976	June 1977
Experimental group II (5)* Hearing loss 81.0 ±24.4 dB	7.3 ±0.7	7.8 ±0.7	13.6 ±5.6	17.0 ±3.5	6.4 ±0.8	5.2 ±1.4
Control group II (7) Hearing loss 72.1 ±14.7 dB	6.9 ±0.5	7.4 ±0.5	12.7 ±3.6	13.7 ±4.7	6.9 ±1.6	5.8 2.0

* Results from only those of group who were recruited in 1975–6.

From *The Lancet*, 21 October 1978, by kind permission.

Reading

The results (Table 4 and Appendix 3, pp. 170–3) for the experimental and control groups (I and II) show a statistically significant improvement in word

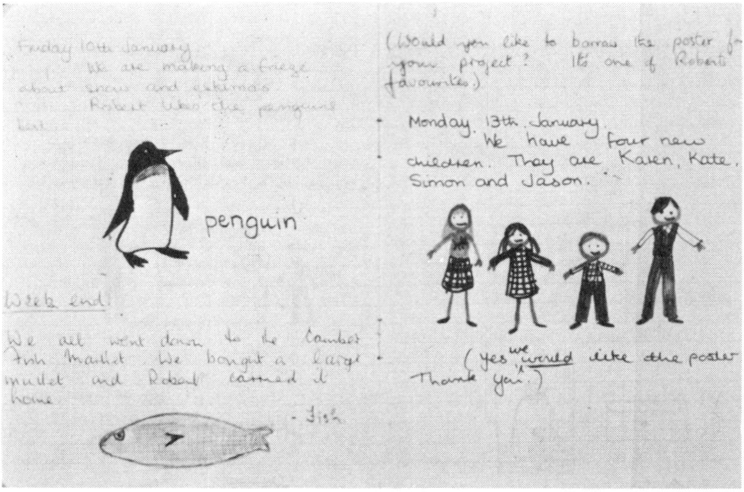
Friday 10th January.
We are making a frieze about snow and eskimos.
Robert likes the penguins best.
penguin
Week end.
We all went down to the Camber Fish Market. We bought a large mullet and Robert carried it home.
fish
(Would you like to borrow the poster for your project? It's one of Robert's favourites.)
Monday. 13th January.
We have four new children. They are Karen, Kate, Simon and Jason.
(Yes we would like the poster Thank you.)

A

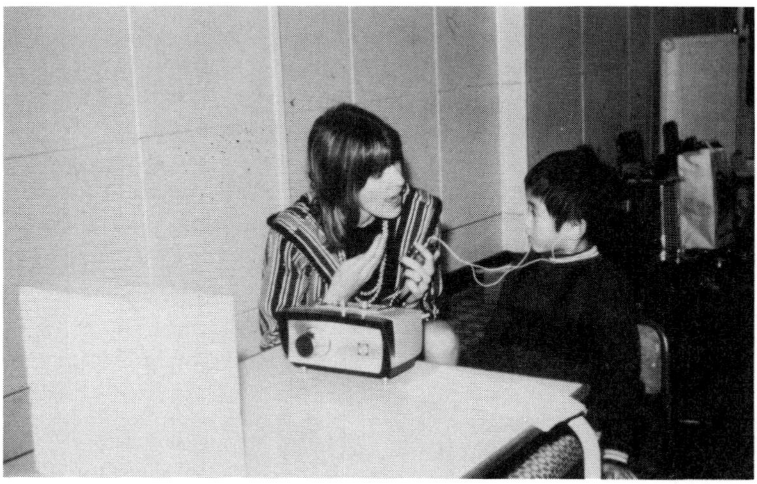

B

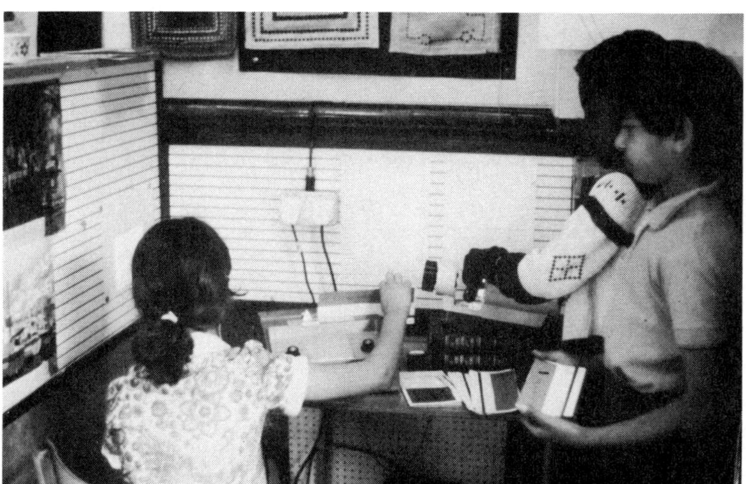

C

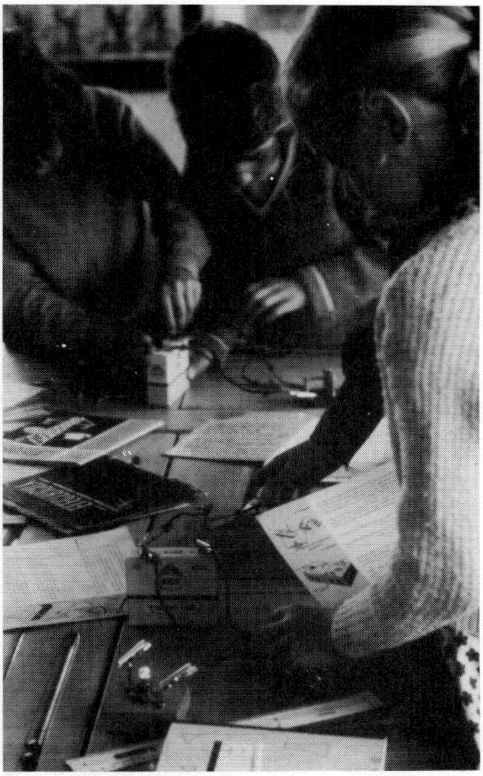

D

Figure 12 Further assistance and growing independence towards the end of the primary school stage.
(a) A home/school notebook.
(b) Cued speech for a child with lip-reading problems. Conventional gestures and basic signs can also be used for certain children without influencing other deaf children's oral education.
(c) Group work using a Language Master and slide projector. (Benefits of regular communication with normally hearing children should never be under-rated.)
(d) A hearing-impaired child can often cope adequately with a card with simplified instructions.

recognition by the former over the latter in each year after the experimental group had left the unit class. (The significance testing was based on 95 per cent confidence intervals.) Reading test scores shown for Experimental Group I are depressed at the upper levels due to the Hamp test having a maximum of 11.0 years. One child in this group scored maximum in 1976 and two in 1977. On Daniels and Diack's Graded Test of Reading Experience,[68] scores of 11.4 years in 1976 and 12.9 and 11.1 years in 1977 were achieved.

The more rapid velocity of progress shown by Experimental Group II children over Control Group II (Table 5) is not significant (by inspection) with such small numbers.

Speech
Both experimental groups achieved better articulation and rate of utterance scores than the control group children. This result is noteworthy in view of the poor patterns of English received in eight of the ten research children's homes.

Teachers
It should be mentioned that staffing in the infant and secondary school units during the 1975–7 school years was also generous: two teachers and two

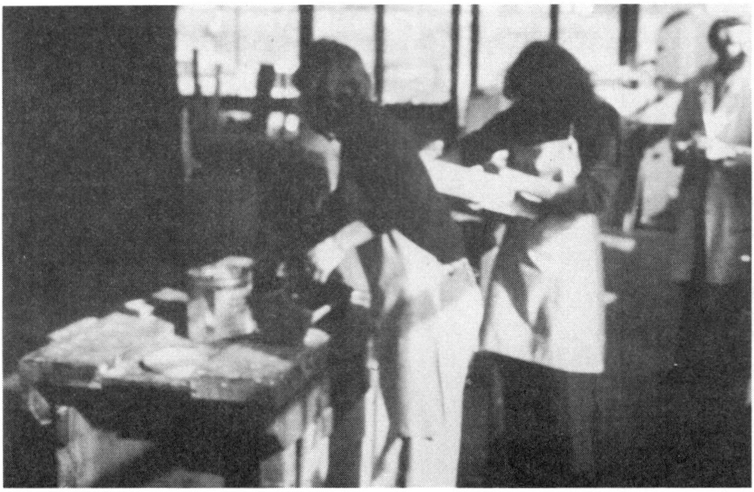

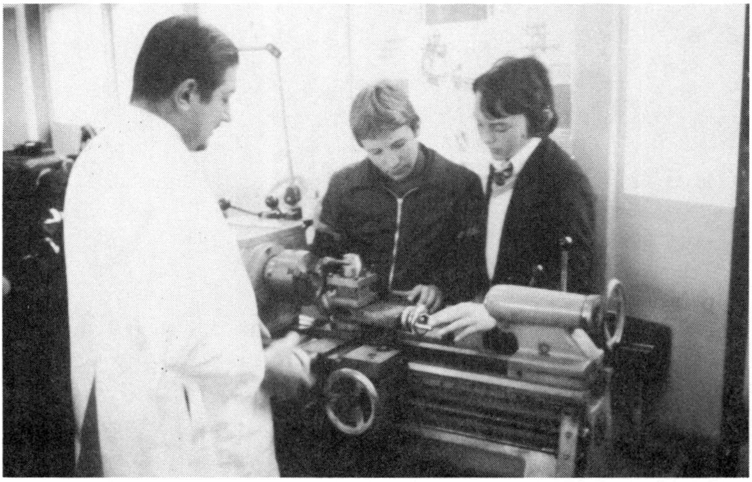

A

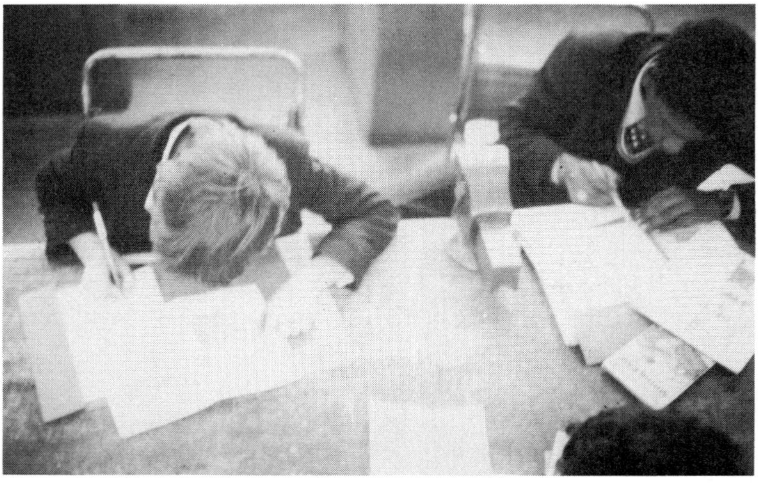

B

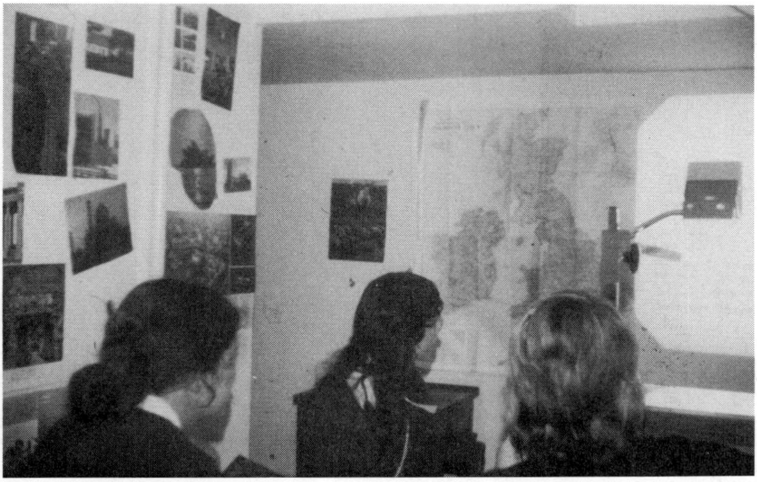

C

Figure 13 At secondary (high) school and tertiary (college) levels, aided individual integration has recently been particularly successful.
(a) Metal and woodworking practice with deaf students in individually integrated situations.
(b) Metal-working theory.
(c) Individual tutoring in social studies for a profoundly deaf 14-year-old girl and a normally hearing student with reading difficulties. (The teacher of the deaf collaborates closely with staff of the ordinary school.)

welfare assistants for ten children, and five teachers for 29 children respectively. In addition, much greater integration into the main school classes (50 per cent at the secondary level) enabled far more individual and small group teaching to be undertaken.

The teacher–pupil ratio in this experiment was approximately one teacher for two children – higher than one would recommend in most other areas, unless there were serious difficulties in addition to the children's hearing handicap, or large distances existing between schools as, for example, in large country authorities. More probable general provision is tentatively suggested in Table 10 (p. 138) with significant reductions in cost which make individual-integration programmes feasible.

The four teachers of the deaf and the six support teachers, who had been associated with this experiment since 1973, had without exception been impressed by the possibilities of this form of educating deaf and partially hearing children. The individual teaching had enabled them to develop close relationships with the children and was felt to have contributed markedly to the success of the scheme. The head teacher of the school for deaf children, after a cautious introductory period, was (and is still) firmly behind the expansion of this project. Head teachers and class teachers of the ordinary schools have expressed their appreciation of the support teaching offered to each research child and also to other children with learning difficulties who have frequently joined them in small group teaching. Genuine interest has existed throughout the four-and-a-half years of this experiment. (In one case, during 1977, a head teacher of a comprehensive school suggested that the support provided for one research child was more than was necessary, and the comment was quite frequently made by teachers and head teachers that 'I've got quite a few others who could do with the sort of help that's being offered that deaf one.')

Parents
In all cases, during each year of this experiment, parents expressed their approval of the fact that their children could attend their local schools and were very pleased with results achieved to date. It was emphasised, however, that in 11 of the 14 cases studied, there had been less parental participation in the educational programmes offered to the children than one would have wished.

The children
One of the original six experimental children left the area after two years, and in July 1975 she was withdrawn from the research group due to frequent truancy from school; for the last ten months she attended the school for deaf children, being called for each day by taxi and attending much more regularly. The head teacher of her comprehensive secondary school was insistent that her poor attendance there was due to social factors rather than any undue strain being placed on her during school hours. (She was a West Indian girl from a broken home and her mother reported that she became involved with some older girls who encouraged her to absent herself from school and 'listen to records'.)

Only one of the present 13 experimental children has ever expressed a wish to return to the unit or school for deaf children, and this was only temporary. All the children now appear to the teachers involved to enjoy their schooling. One child in Experimental Group 1 (hearing loss 95 dB) was reported not to have established any very close friendships, but he *did* have quite easy casual relationships with other members of his form. It is remarkable (and splendid) that *all* of the other 12 children have several close friends who talk and play happily with them each day. The fact that genuine friendships *do* develop between deaf and normally hearing children and young adults when they are individually integrated is one of the most significant findings of the studies reported in this book. It has been well established in much larger studies[65,187] that when *groups* of hearing-impaired students are placed with normally hearing ones, very few close friendships between the two groups ever occur.

By 1977, four of the 13 children in the experimental group all attended the same large comprehensive secondary school which happened to be their neighbourhood school. They were enrolled in different forms and rarely met during school hours. One full-time support teacher was available to these four children and a teacher of the deaf visited each day to assist with speech work and to advise.

General discussion

If head and senior teachers of special schools are expected to develop interest in this new approach, it seems important that they should at least be given professional oversight of these more severely handicapped children when they move out individually into their local ordinary schools, and special schools should be staffed to enable this. This *is* the case in a few areas of England and the United States and in New Zealand but is rarely found elsewhere. Unfortunately, the Warnock Report sees no such role for head teachers of special schools.[232] It is suggested here, however, that local education authority administrators might well consider inviting head teachers to visit their integration programmes from time to time and, if possible, on a regular basis.

In all the individual-integration programmes studied above, friendships with normally hearing children have been shown to develop much more frequently than when deaf children attend units or special schools.[55,187] In addition, in adult education in the United Kingdom and the United States, individual students have successfully attended tutorials and classes at the Open University (UK) and in colleges of further education with appropriate assistance.[18,31,34] It is felt, however, that in adulthood some hearing-impaired people are likely always to need the deaf clubs and societies which have meant so much to so many in the past, especially for relaxed social communication and for spiritual aid.

It has become clear that the child's age, personality, extent of the handicap or handicaps, amount of home support and size of class in the ordinary school can all affect the amount of additional support required for successful individual integration.

Copies of reports on the weekly programmes of two of the experimental children are included as Appendix 4, pages 174–9.

Hearing-impaired children in ordinary schools in Norfolk

Between 1968 and 1979 the policy of educating as many deaf and partially hearing children as possible in ordinary schools was pursued by the Norfolk (UK) Education Authority. By November 1977, 246 of the 301 children in Norfolk issued with hearing aids (81.7 per cent) were attending their local ordinary schools. They received visits from advisory teachers of the deaf as infrequently as twice per term and as often as once each day – depending on the extent of each child's handicap.[173]

During 1977, 22 of the most severely handicapped children in ordinary schools in central, eastern and southern Norfolk were seen by the writer (Table 6). Five children had very severe hearing losses (90+ dB) and the mean for all the 22 children was 73 dB. Reading test results for four of the five children with hearing losses in excess of 90 dB were markedly better than most of those achieved by children enrolled in units in ordinary schools or in schools for deaf children, and their speech intelligibility was rather better. Socially, all but three of these 22 children had made at least one close friendship with a normally hearing child, and *all* had made a number of quite warm casual relationships.

Table 6 Twenty-two Norfolk children individually integrated in their local schools, 1976–7

Child	*Hearing Loss* (Better ear threshold for 500, 1000, 2000 Hz)	*Academic Ability*	*Chron. Age*	*Reading Age*	*Speech (Chap. 10) Cons. Intell.*	*Rate*
1	85	C	13.5	7.6	13	5.5
2	65	C	12.8	9.0	21	4.0
3	65	C−	12.6	8.1	15	3.5
4	55	C−	11.9	10.9	22	5.0
5	80	C	11.1	7.3	20	5.0
6	95	C+	10.9	8.8	20	5.5
7	65	C+	10.0	7.6	19	5.5
8	50	D+	9.4	8.1	15	5.3
9	60	C−	9.2	7.1	20	6.0
10	70	C	9.0	8.5	15	5.6
11	100	C+	8.5	7.5	*Abs.	*Abs.
12	95	C	7.5	8.5	17	5.0
13	80	C+	7.5	6.1	12	8.0
14	70	C−	7.0	6.8	14	6.0
15	95	B+	6.9	7.7	13	6.5
16	70	C	6.8	5.6	18	9.0
17	65	C−	6.5	6.1	19	5.0
18	65	C−	5.5	−5.5	10	2.5
19	90+	C+	5.4	5.7	13	8.5
20	115	B+	4.8	−5.5	2	NA
†21	?(55)	C	6.5	−5.5	2	6.0
22	65	C	4.5	−5.5	10	7.5

* Absent at time of testing others in this area.
† Both ears totally occluded – neurally near normal.

In 16 of these 22 cases, however, considerably more individual assistance was felt to be required if academic achievements were to be maintained and, in many cases, approximate those of normally hearing children of the same mental age levels. Seventeen of the children in the infant, primary and secondary schools' units in Norwich were also tested, and in nearly all cases, their educational and social adjustment results, as in larger studies, gave no cause for complacency (Appendix 5, p. 180).

After full discussions with the teacher of the deaf and the audiologist in charge and his staff, and several consultations with senior administrative officers and the chief psychologist at the Norfolk Education Office, the following plan was evolved in April 1978 to improve the existing individual-integration programme in Norfolk and to monitor it as part of the research in this field. Although, as will be seen later, it was not possible to introduce this plan, brief details are included as it is felt they may be helpful to other education authorities when extending their individual-integration programmes.

The Norfolk plan

Year 1

(1) Move selected children from the first and middle school hearing-impaired units into their own local schools.
(2) Move other children from these units to more integrated situations within these two schools after improving the opportunities for more frequent individual teaching where required.
(3) Offer more tutorial sessions to hearing-impaired children at present enrolled in the comprehensive high school.
(4) Offer more frequent individual assistance to 40 children at present attending their local schools, to ensure the success of the present educational policy.

Year 2

(5) Continue the above studies and, if successful:
(6) consider moving certain carefully selected children who at that time were attending deaf schools and units back into their neighbourhood schools – and provide them with a great deal of individual assistance (*see* chapter 9).
(7) Make a preliminary study of the effect of home assistants – trained by the authority and the National Deaf Children's Society (chapter 9) – working with those parents who were felt to require most guidance and encouragement.

Staffing

(1) Through redeployment of existing staff, it was thought it would have been possible for one teacher of the deaf and one welfare assistant to deal with the needs of the reduced number of children in both the infant and primary school units.
(2) The second teacher of the deaf and the part-time welfare assistant might then have been able to be employed in an itinerant capacity in the Central Area schools.
(3) Additional staffing would have been required to cover the needs of the other research children – it was suggested that three full-time remedial teachers and the equivalent of two full-time welfare assistants (on maximum scale) should be employed in other parts of the county. As is commonly acknowledged, less able children require proportionately more individual assistance. If possible, qualified teachers would have been employed part-time to work as welfare assistants with such children.

Financial (1978 scales)

Teachers of the deaf – no increase			
Remedial assistant teachers	3 × £3,850 (mid point of scale)	=£11,550	
	Plus 5%	578	
		£12,128	
Travel	3 × £400	1,200	
		£13,328	
	for 3 years		=£39,984
Welfare assistants	2 × £2,205 (maximum scale)	=£4,410	
	Plus 5%	225	
		£4,635	
	for 3 years		=£13,905
	Total		£53,889
Half-time research officer, plus insurance, subsistence, travel and test materials for 3 years			£8,469
		Total	£62,358

Although the local education authority agreed to finance both staff and parent training schemes, it was not possible for them to fund the full extension due to the stringent financial climate at that time.

6

A survey of individualised integration in New Zealand 1976

A survey of the itinerant teacher of the deaf service in New Zealand was conducted from January to April 1976 at the request of the Director-General of Education in Wellington. The aim was to assess the value of this new service and make recommendations. Information was gathered using structured interviews of itinerant teachers, advisers, head teachers or heads of departments and class teachers, parents and children (Appendix 6, pp. 181–94).

The report of this survey is included here in considerable detail because the children seen were more severely deaf than those individually integrated in most areas of other countries studied. The amount and type of special education offered each child also varied considerably from one area of New Zealand to another, and these data are felt also to be useful for comparative purposes.

The itinerant teacher service

The itinerant teacher of the deaf service was begun in Auckland in 1971 with one teacher.* By January 1976, nine itinerant teachers had been appointed in various parts of New Zealand, and their main function was to assist individual children from schools for the deaf or units who had transferred to their local ordinary schools. Assistance was given for up to two hours per child per week, and class teachers were assisted in the management of these children.

In the Auckland area, itinerant teachers had divided each school day into four sessions, and thus were able to see up to 18 children individually between Monday morning and lunch-time on Fridays. The teachers spent Friday afternoons at the school for deaf children obtaining teaching materials from the media centre and libraries and, when necessary, discussing cases with the more senior advisory teachers of the deaf.* In Christchurch and Wellington,

* The distinction between *itinerant* and *advisory* teachers of the deaf is discussed in chapter 9.

fewer children were seen each week (Table 7) but more than one visit was made to a number of the children, and sessions, especially for younger children, were usually much shorter than a quarter of each school day.

During the nine weeks of this survey, it was possible to make visits to 40 primary schools, 14 secondary schools and three schools for deaf children. Forty-eight children were seen who had received itinerant teaching in the Auckland, Wellington and Christchurch areas, and six children in Auckland who were receiving tutoring sessions in ordinary schools. The homes of 15 children were visited and the parents of 21 other children were interviewed in the schools.

Table 7 Case loads of five itinerant teachers of the deaf

Itinerant teacher	No. of children	Age range	Average hearing loss
1 Auckland	18	7.3–14.5 years	70.8 dB (teachers 1–3)
2 ,,	17	6.0–16.4 ,,	
3 ,,	18	12.0–15.9 ,,	
4 Wellington	13	6.0–16.8 ,,	76.0 dB
5 Christchurch	12	6.2–16.6 ,,	58.3 dB

All the itinerant teachers seen had established excellent relationships with schools and with parents and children. For example, the head teachers in every case felt that the service was of very considerable value, and teachers frequently commented on how the deaf children had improved as soon as this service was begun. Morale among the itinerant teachers interviewed was high.

Difficulties occurred in a number of cases, however, when the itinerant teachers took children from lessons which were either of great interest to them or which were felt to be important to them. Both children and itinerant teachers frequently commented upon this. Four children were taking speech therapy in addition to receiving itinerant teaching help and, although in two cases, this was very much appreciated because the speech therapist was so capable and stimulating, one wondered about the advisability of disrupting these children's programmes further by going to speech therapy clinics which frequently required missing a large portion of their ordinary timetable. (Teachers of the deaf are, of course, normally expected to teach speech to deaf children.)

As a remedy for this, one remedial teacher in a large residential secondary school in Auckland arranged to meet a partially hearing boy for five minutes before and after school each day to help him overcome difficulties with school work or with his social life, and this was much appreciated by the child and his parents as well as by the itinerant teacher of the deaf.[225]

Virtually all the itinerant teaching was conducted on a one-to-one basis and this was clearly helpful to the children, both academically and personally. From the social integration aspect, however, it was felt that micro-unit teaching would have been beneficial for at least part of these tutoring sessions.

Two or three classmates can frequently engage in reading activities and games which can be enjoyable and beneficial and, at the same time, help to establish the understanding and warm relationships which it is so desirable to foster. One headmaster in Wellington suggested that pairs of children might take it in turn to join the partially hearing child in such activities, and perhaps this method would be worthwhile to enable all class members to speak to and understand the handicapped student better and vice versa. If such small group sessions can be conducted in the main classroom without causing undue disruption, and perhaps using the gain control of a speech-training aid or tradio transmitter aid to reduce extraneous noise, so much the better.

The absence of micro-teaching-unit sessions, the lack of contact with the homes, the need for additional itinerant teaching sessions for many of the children and the absence of speech teaching were the four areas in the role of the itinerant teacher which caused concern. Despite this, the overall view of this new and developing service was encouraging. As will be shown below, only three of the 54 children seen stated that they were not happy in their new schools and only one of these said that she preferred her previous (unit) placement to her present one. In addition, only one child was unable to give the name of a friend made at the present school. Parents, itinerant teachers and the teachers in the ordinary schools were overwhelmingly in favour of this new development in special education.

Enrolments

The enrolments of various schools visited were:

- ★ 8 secondary (high) schools with 364 to 1430 students (mean=963)
- ★ 6 intermediate schools (10- to 11-year-old children) with 540 to 820 students (mean=728.3)
- ★ 41 primary schools with 183 to 512 students (mean=374.4)

The sizes of the classes to which the research children were attached ranged:

- ★ in secondary schools, from 15 to 32 students (mean=29.7)
- ★ in intermediate schools, from 26 to 33 students (mean=29.4)
- ★ in primary schools, from 22 to 41 students (mean=31.3)

These sizes were slightly higher than one might have expected so early in the school year, but were not commented upon by any of the teachers interviewed.

The average length of attendance of the research children in the schools was 1 year 8 months, although one-fifth of the children had been attending their schools for only ten weeks or less. Class teachers, in the main, felt that they knew the research children either 'a little better' or 'much better' than other children in their classes. This was probably due to the attention drawn to them by the itinerant and tutoring teachers, and to the one-day induction course which they had all attended (see below).

Itinerant teacher visits

As mentioned earlier, in the Auckland area each child was visited once a week, and these visits were usually of a quarter of a day's duration. In Wellington and Christchurch, only 13 and 12 children, respectively, were being seen by the itinerant teachers, and in most cases two and occasionally three visits were being made to each child. Class teachers considered that one-third of this group of children were receiving adequate support from the itinerant teachers; the remainder were felt to require one or two more visits each week. In five cases - two in Auckland, two in Wellington and one in Christchurch - four or five visits each week were felt to be necessary, so great was the children's handicap.

Severity of educational handicap

It is interesting to note that only one-third of these deaf and partially hearing children had educational handicaps which the class teachers rated as more severe than those of some other members of their classes. Twelve had educational handicaps which were 'about the same' as those of some other class members; the problems of 17 were 'not so severe'; and five hearing-impaired children had handicaps which were considered 'not nearly so severe'.

Need for such remedial teaching of other children

This varied a great deal depending on the area visited. In a depressed, high-immigrant area in Auckland, for example, one head teacher felt that three-quarters of his school would profit from some such individual assistance (see Glynn[103]). In a well-to-do area of Christchurch, on the other hand, another head teacher of a large primary school felt that none of the children needed such intensive therapy. Overall, however, only five of the 47 teachers consulted felt that no children needed such help - in six classes one-third of the children were considered in need of remedial assistance. An average of five children in each class were felt by the class teachers interviewed to need remedial assistance.

The question whether such remedial teaching was needed was asked for two reasons:

(1) to ascertain whether a *remedial teacher* attached to many of the schools might be able to assist the hearing-impaired child and then help others within the same school who had hearing difficulties. This, of course, would eliminate the travelling between schools which can be expensive, time-consuming and irksome.

(2) to assay the possibility of itinerant teachers conducting remedial work in micro-teaching units as well as individually (the case at present). Although the purpose of such small group teaching in this case would be primarily for social purposes, there are also valid educational (and even political) reasons for adopting this type of teaching. All but a handful of the head teachers

interviewed were most interested in the possibility of any such remedial assistance, but all recognised the problem created by the prevailing economic stringency.

None of the itinerant teachers normally taught hearing children with the deaf ones, but in two cases (in Wellington and Christchurch), they did teach groups or whole classes occasionally – telling or reading them stories and so on. This was very much appreciated by both the children and the teachers.

Attitudes towards the itinerant teacher service

Of all the 73 head and class teachers interviewed, only one said she felt that the itinerant service was 'of doubtful value'. Fifty-two were 'very much in favour' of it, and a further 20 believed it to be 'probably quite useful' (and a number of these said this because they 'did not know the service well enough yet'). This finding was felt to be a tribute to those who had selected the itinerant teachers, and to the conscientious, tactful and imaginative ways in which most of these teachers worked.

It was clear that advisory teachers, after setting up the itinerant teaching service, did not take an active part in teaching the children or advising their teachers or parents. This was felt to be understandable when advisers had such heavy caseloads of other children.

Interviews with the children

Twenty-three of the children interviewed said that they could only understand the teacher in class 'sometimes', 12 said 'often' and nine 'usually'. It was not always clear whether the lack of comprehension was due to not being able to hear what was being said or to a lack of understanding. It was probably a combination of both, but it *does* emphasise that many of these children were missing a great deal in oral class lessons. Notes as included in chapter 9 can be useful to class teachers (pp. 131–3).

It was encouraging that three-quarters of the group said they liked their present school and only three of the children said that they did not like it. The remainder said that school was 'all right'. It is interesting that only one child said that she would prefer to go back to the unit or school for deaf children.

Three children said that they did not like itinerant teaching, and a further 12 that they liked it 'a little'. The remainder (about two-thirds) said they liked these visits 'quite a lot' or 'very much'.

One reason why nearly a third of the group seemed somewhat diffident about itinerant teaching help was that (a) they did not wish to be isolated from their classmates, and (b) they liked the help but, that as a result, they missed work being done by the rest of the class. For example, one boy said, 'Last Thursday I missed English and on Friday we had a test and I got a very low mark.' (When it was suggested that perhaps some itinerant teaching could be arranged during a lunch-time, this boy replied, 'No – because I must have my lunch!') (See 'Recommendations for Itinerant Teachers', numbers 7, 8, 9, 11, 12 and 15.)

The commonest reason for wanting the visits was that they 'help me with my work', and a number of the children were careful to take their difficulties to the itinerant teachers. (As a reason for liking the visits 'very much', one girl said, 'You see, I miss maths, and I *hate* maths.')

With regard to the deaf children's ability to form friendships with normally hearing children, some explanation of the data in Table 8 is necessary. All the 38 research children questioned about this said that they had at least one friend in class and this was encouraging. It must be said, however, that not all the normally hearing children reciprocated. If time had permitted, it would have been interesting to have seen to what extent the handicapped children were regarded as 'best friends' by their normally hearing classmates.

Table 8 Deaf children's 'best friends' among normally hearing children

						Total
(a) In class:	6	research children named	1	best friend in their class		6
	10	,, ,, ,,	2	,, friends ,, ,, ,,		20
	12	,, ,, ,,	3	,, ,, ,, ,, ,,		42
	6	,, , ,,	4	,, ,, ,, ,, ,,		24
	2	,, ,, ,,	5	,, ,, ,, ,, ,,		10
	36					102

					Total
(b) At home:	6	research children named	no	best friends at home	0
	14	,, ,, ,,	1	,, friend ,, ,,	14
	7	,, ,, ,,	3	,, friends ,, ,,	14
	7	,, ,, ,,	3	,, ,, ,, ,,	21
	2	,, ,, ,,	4	,, ,, ,, ,,	16
	36				65

Fewer normally hearing friends were claimed by the research children at home, but this was considered natural since many children play mainly with their siblings there. Only ten of the 38 hearing-impaired children who had best friends at school named the same children as best friends at home. Again, this is not surprising, since even when children attend the same class, their homes may be inconveniently far away from one another. The record of friendships, however, was far better than was the case in the study made of children attending three units in ordinary schools in England in 1970–1.[65] In that case, it will be remembered (chapter 2), only three of the 64 children claimed a best friend among the normally hearing children, and they were living so far apart that no contact was possible after school or at weekends.

Reading and speech assessments

Reading

Two tests were used: the Daniels and Diack Graded Test of Reading Experience[68] and Hamp's Picture-Assisted Reading Test[107] (*see* chapter 10, pp. 152–4). Due to the high correlation between these (0.963) both sets of results were combined in the overall assessment of these children's reading ability. In some cases, due to last minute changes in the schools' timetables, unexpected delays in interviewing children, parents or teachers and so on, it was not possible to administer either reading test.

These were felt to contain a representative sample of the children individually integrated into ordinary schools who were receiving regular special teaching.

Although the reading ages placed nearly all of these children in the 'retarded reader' category,* there was no evidence that the velocity of their progress in the present situation is less than in their earlier placement in units or schools for deaf children. This should, of course, be carefully monitored in future. A number of comments from both parents and itinerant teachers suggested that many of the children were applying themselves to their studies more rigorously than ever before and it is to be hoped that this enthusiasm can be maintained.

Low academic achievement and retarded speech and language development are by no means uncommon in the education of deaf and partially hearing children.[46,83,228,235] It was recommended that every effort should be made to overcome these deficiencies, and the conclusion of this writer was that an increase of a variety of forms of such itinerant teaching was most likely to achieve the most satisfactory educational and social results.

The hearing losses of the itinerant teaching group were mainly in the 'severe', but not 'profound' category. Despite intelligence ratings which were negatively skewed, no child had obtained a reading age in excess of his or her chronological age nor speech which could be rated as 'normal'. This, of course, emphasises the serious effect of deafness upon communication skills which has been noted in most other studies. It would, however, be of great interest to ascertain whether the rate of progress in reading and speech was accelerating or decelerating as a result of the individual placement.

Speech

The speech of most of the children gave no cause for complacency. It was suggested that every effort should be made to improve the intelligibility of their speech since they were now in an excellent situation to use oral language and to make the most of any assistance given (*see* Recommendation 12, p. 162). Time did not permit a thorough investigation of each child's speech, and ratings were made of the speech as a result of the interview with each child.

---

* Reading ages greater than two years below chronological ages.

The overall results are felt to be reasonably accurate, but individual ratings should be treated with caution.

Interviews with parents

The parents of 36 of the children were interviewed (15 in their homes and 21 in the children's schools).

It was thought important to seek information about the relationship of the handicapped children to their siblings.

2 children had no siblings.
14 children had 1 sibling (of whom 8 were younger and 6 were older).
9 children had 2 siblings (of whom 9 were younger and 9 were older).
2 children had 3 siblings (all 6 were younger).
2 children had 4 siblings (of whom 5 were younger and 3 were older).
2 children had 5 siblings (of whom 5 were younger and 5 were older).
3 children had 6 siblings (of whom 14 were younger and 4 were older).
1 child had 7 siblings (of whom 6 were younger and 1 was older).
1 child had 8 siblings (of whom 6 were younger and 2 were older).

When the parents were asked about the help that these other children were to their deaf or partially hearing brothers or sisters, seven replied that the brothers and/or sisters were of little assistance, three because they had left home. Ten said that the siblings were of considerable assistance and 16 replied that they were of great assistance.

In five cases, parents reported that their normally hearing children were of tremendous help when they were younger, but not so much now. The siblings seemed to help most by teaching the deaf children games and helping with homework, in shops and in the playground. Two parents stated that their children did not seem to like the deaf child particularly, but that they would 'defend them against other children' if ever this was needed. (Interesting studies by Clay *et al.*[40] have indicated that rivalry and friction between close, normally hearing siblings are extremely common.)

When asked about the degree of difficulty experienced by their children before and after itinerant assistance was given, parents' replies indicated that there was rather less difficulty after the child entered the integration programme than before. Only three of the 36 parents who replied to the question regarding the degree of difficulty experienced by the child *now* stated that there was 'a great deal'. Nine parents considered that their child was still having 'considerable difficulty' and 13 that their child was having 'a little difficulty'. No fewer than 11 parents considered that there were no particular difficulties.

Eighteen parents said 'yes', ten said 'no', and eight 'perhaps' when asked if there was a need for more itinerant assistance. A number of the parents who indicated 'no' or 'perhaps' to this query said that they did not wish their child to miss any more schooling. This point had been raised earlier by children and teachers, and is clearly of importance.

One's expectations as to subject preferences were upheld, and it would be interesting to compare them with those of normally hearing boys and girls. Subjects liked most included art, pottery, sport, dressmaking, ballroom dancing, photography, television lessons, drawing, typing, physical education and social studies. However, four children chose mathematics, three chose spelling, and four chose reading as their favourite subjects. Subjects liked least included English, new mathematics, spelling and book-keeping.

Out of school, parents reported similar activities to the children's likes and dislikes in school, but also included, under 'liked doing most', listening to pop records (played very loudly!), surfing, swimming, playing outdoors, visiting museums, collecting shells, educational toys and playing with dolls. One nine-year-old girl was said to like most 'helping Dad mend the car – it's like an operating theatre!' Activities children liked doing least included: washing the dishes, maths, reading, homework generally, Girl Guides (in one case), housework (six children).

It was thought to be critically important to ascertain whether these handicapped children could make and maintain close friendships. It is considered fundamental that a child should at least be able to feel comfortable while he or she is attending school and that all educational programmes should be carefully monitored to ensure that this is so.

Twenty-three children were reported by their parents to have made close friendships at school – in most cases with two or three children, but in some cases only one. Five parents reported that their children had made friendships with other boys and girls but that these were not really close. Only in one case of the 29 did parents state that a child had no close friends at school. From my own observations and interviews with class and itinerant teachers, some of these parents' ratings on friendships should be treated with caution. At home, 16 of the 29 children whose parents were interviewed had made close friends, three had no friends apart from their brothers and sisters, and seven had acquaintances which could not be described as 'really close friends'.

Over half the group were said to read quite often or a great deal at home. Favourite free reading was chosen from comics, jokes and light books, television advertisements, Golden Books, children's books containing 'lots of direct speech', Cinderella, the *Secret Seven* (Enid Blyton), colourfully illustrated children's books and adventure stories.

Fifteen parents who were asked this question heard their children read every night or nearly every night. Eleven parents helped their children occasionally and four said they never helped them. (Again, these parents' ratings may be somewhat inaccurate as other studies have shown they can be over-optimistic.)[60] Nineteen children belonged to the local library.

It was disappointing that 27 of the parents stated that they had never kept a family diary[51] (several did say, 'but I will do so now').

The following suggestions (not in any particular order) for improving the itinerant teacher service were given by the parents:

* Try to arrange the itinerant service at times when it would least upset the school day. One mother said that her child was most disturbed because he had to miss swimming.
* Home/school notebooks[51] are excellent: 'The class teacher fills ours in daily and it's marvellous really'; 'I have a home/school notebook between me and *both* teachers – it's excellent.'
* More contact required between home and teachers.
* Eight parents said, 'School books should be brought home from time to time.' One said, 'I've never been shown what to do about school work.'
* 'Try not to single the deaf child out too much. Mrs Keir is ideal – she joins in with the class and is just one of the group.'
* Could help be given, as for blind children, in examinations? For example, perhaps a little extra time could be given, and if possible particular care be taken in the wording of questions to help ensure that the deaf child understands what is required.
* A Chinese mother, through an interpreter, said, 'I'd quite like the itinerant teacher to come home after school to help with reading and so on.'
* Could extra tutoring be given for children taking public examinations?
* Could correspondence school* lessons be used for some subjects – biology, for example? (Correspondence school lessons have filled in many of the gaps.)[118,156,237]
* 'I think more help is needed in the problems of social training of deaf children' (mother of ten-year-old deaf child).
* One itinerant teacher was preferred to another because 'She let Jocelyn "side-track" more.'
* Could the children be kept out of classes where the work is way above their heads?
* 'I've arranged private coaching for my child': this from three parents who were convinced that their children were not receiving sufficient support from the present amount of itinerant teaching.
* 'I've noticed she needs the help and responds immediately to the one-to-one approach.'
* 'Is there a possibility of group therapy rather than individual tuition for these children?' (using normally hearing children to make up the group).

Further comments which were made during parent interviews included:

* 'I'm sorry there's no opportunity for the children to learn to take driving licence examinations as was done at the deaf school.'
* 'If mothers don't learn to talk and keep talking, then I think the child is lost.'

---

* Correspondence schools have been set up in the Soviet Union, Norway, Australia and New Zealand and elsewhere to assist children who are unable to attend school owing to ill health or to living in remote country areas.[70,118] In New Zealand, lessons in all school subjects are sent out every two weeks to the parents of these children. The work is marked by teachers back at the correspondence school and the next instalment sent. Assignments are attractively laid out and illustrated, and have been found useful for deaf children in ordinary schools – especially if a support teacher or welfare assistant is available to help (*see* Appendix 12).

- ★ 'I'm determined to take an interest in all that is going on at this school – I didn't at the previous one.'
- ★ 'At school, teachers frequently say "How lovely she is." This is nice, but I also want them to tell me what she needs most – I want the "nitty-gritty".'
- ★ 'He's joined lots of clubs' (since enrolling at the ordinary high school).
- ★ 'He didn't like the long bus ride to the unit. Now he can walk to school and he's much happier.'
- ★ The mother of a 15-year-old, severely deaf, 'strong willed' girl commented: 'Her sisters have more influence over her than I do. I say to them, for example, "Come on girls, can you help me stop Rachel's I'm-going-to-leave-school attitude?" – and they do!'
- ★ 'My boy was minded three times in all his early life, and those three people never offered again.' (This is discussed in some detail later.)
- ★ 'She voluntarily spends hours and hours on workbooks.' (This intelligent, severely deaf, 15-year-old girl was now stimulated by the language-filled environment which surrounded her.)
- ★ 'Ailsa will often lie on her bed for two hours *reading the dictionary*! She never did that sort of thing before.' (A bright 14-year-old, profoundly deaf girl.)
- ★ 'I still remember the tremendous importance of the visiting [advisory] teachers' visits when she was young' (mother of a 15-year-old girl).
- ★ 'His brothers and sisters have been a great help – especially for bringing friends to the house.'
- ★ 'If David [eight-years-old] misses something on the television, Andrew [five-years-old] repeats a great deal.'
- ★ 'The other children help Maudie, and she helps *them*!'
- ★ 'At church the other day, she saw three children in one family and they all had hearing aids. She was delighted to see them.' (See Parents' Recommendation 5, p. 92)
- ★ 'There should be a closer tie up between the school and the home. She didn't know what she was missing to begin with' (a 15-year-old, severely deaf girl).

Parents' recommendations

(1) Itinerant teachers should establish the closest possible relationship with parents.[91] Home/school notebooks between parent and itinerant teacher (and, where possible, class teachers), home visits, and regular telephone calls all help to promote a consistent team approach to overcoming each child's difficulties more effectively.

(2) Consideration should be given to the possibility of groups of two or three mothers collaborating to act as teachers' aides (or 'welfare assistants' as they are called in the United Kingdom) for one another's deaf children. (This might be on the basis of one, two, three or four days or half-days each week, depending on the severity of the children's handicaps. The possibility of this being undertaken voluntarily should be considered if funding such a

scheme by the Department of Education or the Parents' Associations is difficult.)

(3) Similarly, suitably qualified parents might act as tutors to deaf children in secondary schools. If sufficient tutoring time could be made available, some deaf children (and perhaps one or two normally hearing ones) could then be withdrawn for all lessons in a subject – e.g., English or history – and could pursue courses recommended and supervised by itinerant teachers or advisers.

(4) A home-assistants scheme should be examined (*see* chapter 9) to ascertain whether parents of older deaf and partially hearing children can be given the opportunity to assist parents of younger children both at home and at school on a regular basis.

(5) Occasional small meetings between hearing-impaired children should be arranged at which both parents and children can relax and discuss mutual problems and successes. This is particularly important, of course, where children are having difficulty in establishing satisfactory friendships outside school.

Interviews with itinerant teachers

Itinerant teachers were asked to fill in six forms covering 'a representative sample' of six of the individual children for whom they were responsible (*see* Appendix 6, pp. 181–2). A total of 30 questionnaires were returned and these are analysed below.

Only one child in eight had been observed in his or her classroom, although three itinerant teachers said that they would like to do this. Some explained that, as it was early in the school year, they had not pressed the matter.

None of the 30 children was felt by the teachers of the deaf to be receiving 'too much time'; 13 were receiving 'sufficient time'; ten, 'not quite enough'; and seven, 'not nearly enough'. This was felt to be a finding of considerable significance and was confirmed by the writer's own observations, interviews and discussions, and by the test results.

Revision of work given by the class teacher included social studies, science, discussions of centres of interest, mathematics (eight children) and mathematics vocabulary (five children). English grammar and syntax were mentioned frequently – for example, unfamiliar vocabulary, spelling, language skills, word endings, punctuation and finding the main idea in a paragraph.

Work which was introduced by the itinerant teacher included pre-teaching of social studies topics (12 children), initial work with phonics, vocabulary building, reading stories, tape-recording conversations and replaying them (seven- and 11-year-old children with hearing losses of 70 dB), diary writing, general knowledge and discussions.

The relationship between the itinerant teacher and the class teacher was considered to be very close in 12 cases, close in five cases, and not very close in 13 cases. In eight of the latter group, teachers explained that since it was so early in the year only two or three visits had been made to the school. Two in Auckland mentioned that the relationship would improve after the one-day course for head and class teachers to be held at the school for deaf children early in the second month of the school year. This involved talks on the medical and educational aspects of deafness, video tapes of deaf children being taught, and hearing a tape recording of filtered speech which illustrated the effect of different degrees of hearing loss very effectively.

It was disappointing that half these 30 children were felt to be receiving little educational help from home. It was not, however, considered correct by the heads of the schools for deaf children that itinerant teachers should visit homes, and in only six cases had visits been made.

At the infant and primary level, the following books were felt to have been useful: Scott Foresman *Basic Readers; McKee Readers; Think and Do* books; *Living Things; Oxford Colour Readers;* the *New Zealand Reading Handbook; Recreational Reading; Thorndike Junior Dictionary;* Richard Scarry's and Dr Seuss' illustrated dictionaries (for children up to eight years of age).

At the secondary level, books included: the *New Reading* series (12-year-olds); *Let's Make English Live* series; Tin-Tin books; *Scholastic Readers;* adventure stories; animal stories; Department of Education readers; *Thorndike Dictionary*; atlases; *The Tutor System* (MIT Press), check lists of everyday phrases and colloquialisms; 'The home/school notebooks have been very helpful.' (*See* Dale.)[24,56]

Miscellaneous points included:

* 'An hour and a half is too long for one teaching session.'
* 'There is no routine in one class and the deaf child seems lost when I go there in the mornings.'
* 'The six- and eight-day timetables in intermediates (middle schools) and high schools create problems for itinerant teaching.'
* 'One mother was asked to help with her daughter's reading, but she said, "I used to, but it always ended in fighting so I gave up".'
* 'We often don't cover the amount of work set by the class teacher.'

The five itinerant teachers filled in one further questionnaire (*see* Appendix 6, p. 183) regarding their training for this new teaching post and their feelings about their work. Replies are summarised below.

Training for itinerant teaching consisted of one week with advisers (peripatetic teachers of the deaf); the itinerant teachers were also given children's files to study and made a school visit, but not a home visit, to each child.

The teachers were asked whether any specialist training was necessary. One itinerant teacher felt that work in a school for deaf children developed sympathy for the children. Four felt that some training in deaf teaching was required for those itinerant teachers dealing with younger, very deaf children. To help the partially hearing and the high school children, however, full specialist training courses for teachers of the deaf were not considered necessary. (It will be remembered that support for this view was given in the Milan integration service – *see* chapter 4, p. 41.)

Additional training which was felt to be needed included:

* More speech work.
* Work in both a school for deaf children and an ordinary school.

* A three- to four-day course in language teaching and remedial work.
* A period of observation of itinerant teachers would be ideal.
* Guidance in public relations techniques.
* Knowledge of the attainments of the whole class so that the deaf child's progress could be measured.
* A study of the present writer's books and publications.
* A thorough knowledge of what is available in the school for the deaf library and media centre.
* More emphasis on handicapped children at teachers' colleges.

Four itinerant teachers felt that the work was 'very satisfying' and the other two 'satisfying'. 'I love it,' said one. 'By the end of the second term I get fed up – but I still love it.' Another reported that 'Two to three years seems a reasonable time to stay in this work,' while two teachers said: 'I'd be happy to keep doing this work until I retire.'

Points made regarding administrative aspects of the work included:

* 'It's important to relate closely to the advisory teachers of the deaf.'
* 'It is difficult to work closely with a class teacher if you don't have her programme' (or if she doesn't *have* a programme).
* 'I always go to the classroom to pick up the child and this gives the class teacher a chance to speak to me.'
* 'We have been told [by the school for the deaf] not to telephone the parents, but I have found that parent–class teacher–itinerant teacher collaboration is really possible and it works well.'
* 'Last year I tried notebooks for each class teacher, so he or she could let me know of work required by them of me, but it didn't work because most preferred to communicate orally with me.' Another teacher, however, commented, 'Ten (out of 15) give me lists of work covered. They're not always accurate though; for example, some children already knew the work that had been taught.'
* 'I think it's important to let the teachers know that you're on the same level – in other words, we're not advisers or inspectors. I used to say to them, "I'm a teacher of the deaf from the deaf school, but I have had a class of 42 five-year-olds in an ordinary school, and I know that people like myself can be a nuisance – you'll forget I'm coming sometimes, but don't worry about it. We are both necessary to help this deaf boy (or girl)." ' I used the classroom programme as the basis and backed things up with material from the media centre and library at the deaf school. 'The children very very rarely forgot that I was coming – and this was encouraging to me.' (This itinerant teacher had been extremely successful in her work.)

Other suggestions, observations and comments included:

* 'Young teachers, just out of college, are best for our children.' (This observation was made on another occasion by three bright, normally hearing children, and when asked why, they replied, 'Young teachers *listen* to us more.')
* 'Things go like a house on fire after the day course at the school for the

deaf.' 'All teachers – heads as well as class teachers – should go to the one-day course at the deaf school.' (*See above*.)

- ⋆ 'I deplore this "he's doing well – after all he's deaf" attitude. I feel we've got to accept the child, understand him, and *extend* him – otherwise we'll get nowhere.'
- ⋆ 'Occasionally I take a story or maths group for the teacher.'
- ⋆ 'If you're having an off day, it's often difficult to appear cheerful and animated – but we must try.'
- ⋆ 'Salaries should be scaled up to a slightly more advanced level, because we *do* give advice to teachers.'
- ⋆ 'It's important to check the hearing aids every time I visit.'
- ⋆ 'I always write a note of what I've done and I give it to the teacher personally.'
- ⋆ 'Schools are good about letting me know if a child is absent and I can then give another child an extra visit.'
- ⋆ 'I always take a book that is round about the child's reading level from the deaf school library and often the class teachers ask me for three or four more!'

Itinerant teachers' recommendations

(1)–(5) As for parents' recommendations (pp. 91–2).

(6) More frequent visits should be made to the children who require help most. [As indicated elsewhere in this book, broadly speaking, younger children of lower intelligence, greater hearing loss and less supporting homes require most additional assistance.]

(7) Visits could be of shorter duration in a number of cases, say, two or three visits of half an hour rather than one visit of one-and-a-quarter or one-and-a-half hours.

(8) Maximum use should be made, for itinerant teaching, of the periods from 8.30–9.30 a.m. each day (i.e., before school begins), as has been achieved in the case of some of the children.

(9) No doubt less popular, but perhaps worth considering, is the possibility of some individual half-hour teaching sessions on Saturday mornings. Teachers would, of course, need equivalent time off during the week – say, on Friday afternoons or Monday mornings. The aim again, as in Recommendation 8, is to provide remedial work at a time which will not interfere with the ordinary school programme. [A certain number of normally hearing children in England *do* have coaching sessions on Saturday mornings and a large number have music lessons.]

(10) The employment of part-time tutors (after, say, a two-week induction period) should be considered for assisting the children who are least handicapped by deafness (hearing losses not in excess of 80 dB in the better ear). This, of course, would allow the itinerant teachers of the deaf to spend more time with the most seriously handicapped children who, at present, require considerably more assistance – both educationally and socially.

(11) Where possible, itinerant teachers should work in the children's class-

rooms – or at least visit the rooms as often as possible to befriend the ordinary children and become known as a teacher as well as just 'the hearing aid lady'.
(12) Home visits should be made briefly but as frequently as possible. [In the writer's experience, the friendly but purposeful 'pop-in' variety of visit does an immense amount of good for parents and children, and also, of course, for the teacher.]
(13) Speech improvement should be one basic aim of every individual session with every child. Regular use of the listening–reading–speaking method,[56,92] as shown in Figure 10 (a), above, as well as some phonetic and phonological work,[31,109,195] as shown in Figure 9 (a) above, should be conducted. Results of successful production of colloquial phrases and words should be sent to parents and class teachers as soon as they are firmly established (*see* Figure 14 (a), below). Records of tests and tape recordings could well be kept for each child.
(14) If it is accepted that itinerant teachers are often required to give guidance to teachers as well as parents (*see* Figure 10 (a), above), and that they could be asked to work from 8.30–9.00 a.m. each day, there seems some justification for readvertising these positions at a somewhat higher level and asking the present incumbents to reapply for them if they so desired. (It is believed that most of them would do so.)
(15) Where possible, opportunities should be created for itinerant teachers to involve one or two of the child's classmates for, say, a third of each session. The purpose of this is partly educational, but primarily social.

Tutoring of children

In the Auckland area, the school for deaf children had arranged for six academically able boys and girls (mean hearing loss 90.00 dB; standard deviation 17.31 dB) to attend their local secondary schools while receiving two hours of individual tutoring help from ordinary school teachers each week. The children had academic ability ratings of A or B on a five-point scale, and an average age of 14.72 years and a reading age (Daniels and Diack Test 12) of 11.8 years. It was possible to interview all six children and speak to their teachers and parents.

Class teachers, form tutors and head teachers, again, were pleased with the attitude of the deaf children, but were sometimes too ready to accept work from them which was of a low standard.

Both children and parents, without exception, commented favourably on the new school placement, but all six children, naturally enough, found some subjects difficult – especially the more verbal ones. English, history and mathematics were, in consequence, common subjects chosen for additional tutoring.

The problem of arranging additional supporting work without interrupting the timetable unduly, and thus jeopardising attainments in other subjects or missing them completely, was in every tutor's mind. Fortunately, three comments arose that seemed of considerable significance.

(1) One tutor, who helped a child for one hour twice each week, commented: 'I find that an hour is a long time.' The implication here was that simply discussing difficulties with the children in a one-to-one, face-to-face situation could become boring for both parties, if not actually counterproductive.
(2) A form tutor at the Penrose High School recommended strongly that tutoring should be done *before* school. When asked whether teachers could be expected to work so early, she replied that, at that school, it was the policy for all teachers to come to work early – 'There are two staff meetings a week at 8.25 a.m. for example.' Teachers were not expected to stay after school, however. These teachers were convinced that before school was a much better time for intensive teaching than after school, when a child might be missing games or clubs and was quite often fatigued.
(3) Another tutor had found it most successful to break her two hours of tutoring into four sessions of half an hour each, and these were conducted before school. A normally hearing friend of the deaf child, who also needed a little extra help, came with her to these. The arrangement seemed to be highly successful.

It was recommended, that
(1) Whenever possible, hearing-impaired children should be offered tutoring before school on four or five days each week.
(2) Where possible, one or two friends, or children living near the handicapped child's home, who needed extra help might be invited to attend. In this way friendships which develop during these sessions might be carried over to after-school hours and weekends.
(3) Parents of the children, and their class teachers, should contact the tutors and advisers regularly to advise and encourage one another.
(4) Where children's handicaps are more severe, more individual tuition was needed and this should, of course, be arranged (at the least disruptive times) during the school day.
(5) Advisory teachers of the deaf should be responsible for training the tutors, visiting them at least once each month to encourage and advise them further, and *annually* administering the educational, audiological and social tests and schedules necessary. The results of the annual educational and social evaluations should be used primarily to compare the velocity of each child's progress with his or her previous achievements.

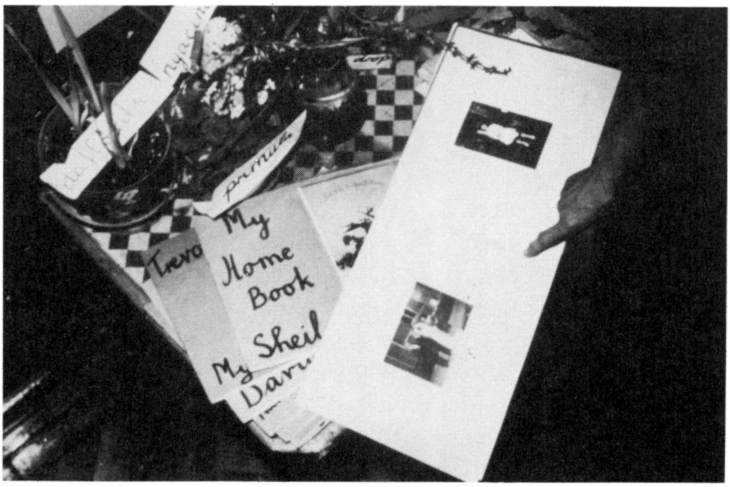

A

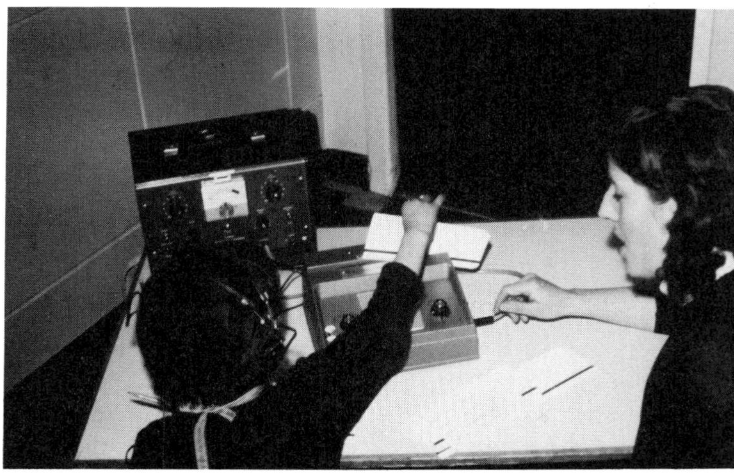

B

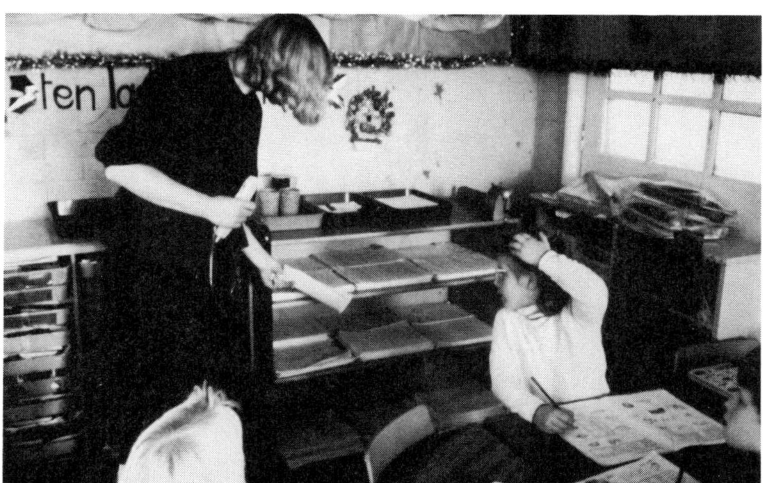

C

D

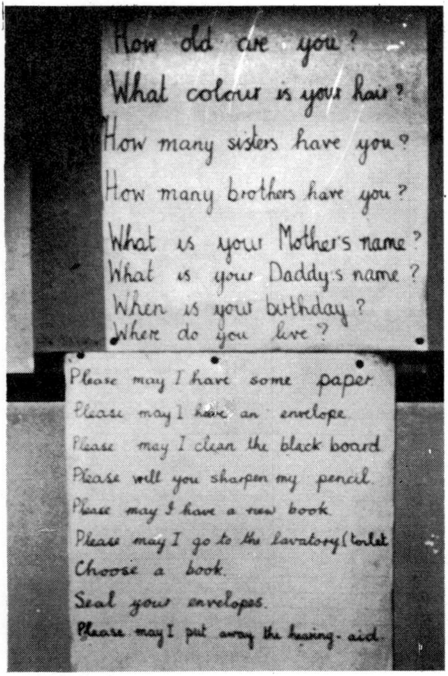

E

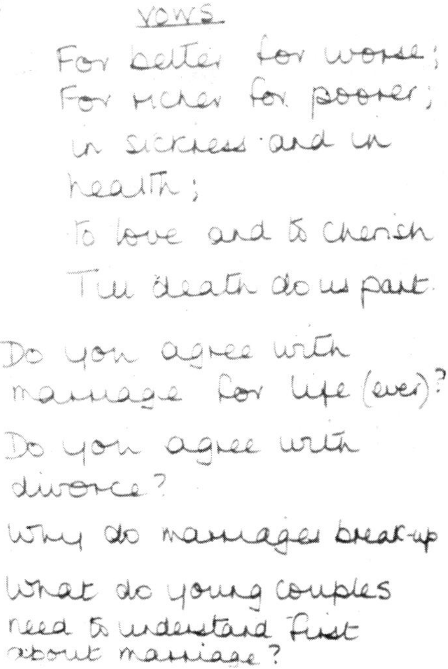

F

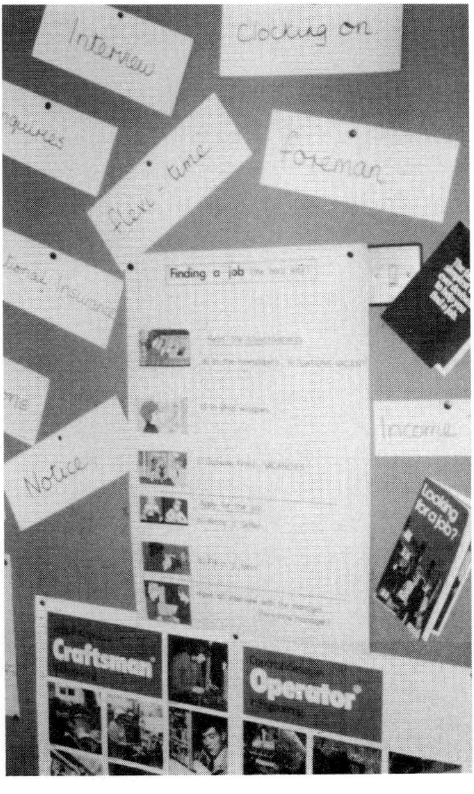

Figure 14 Methods found useful by teachers of the deaf and ordinary school teachers can frequently be exchanged.
(a) Photographs from home can make excellent discussion material for visitors.
(b) Language Masters are excellent for listening and reading exercises, individually or in small groups.
(c) A teacher of the deaf uses mathematics handouts made by the teacher of the ordinary class.
(d) Language forms used frequently by teachers of the deaf can be written on wall charts.
(e) Cards made by a teacher of the deaf and used for discussions with adolescents.
(f) A teacher of the deaf amplifies commercially-produced charts.

7

Integration in developing countries

As indicated earlier, it is now considered urgent that individual-integration programmes in Developing Countries should be given serious consideration. There are, in fact, a large number of handicapped children already attending their local ordinary schools (although often with minimal individual attention) simply because there are no special schools available.[1] Many others, however, live at home and receive no special education at all.[8] The cost of building and administering special day and residential schools has meant that governments of many developing countries have, to date, made only token efforts in this field.[69]

The fact that a growing number of workers in the developed countries[234] have also begun to question whether segregated special educational provision is able adequately to meet the needs of most handicapped children and their families, has begun to cause a number of administrators to consider alternatives.[48,52,86,103,220] In India, for example, the government stated in 1980 that it was now their policy to provide integrated education for as many handicapped children as possible. In Kenya, units in ordinary schools were introduced in the 1960s in preference to special schools. Mexico and Pakistan are currently considering units and individual programmes as alternatives to special schools for many of their deaf children.

Quite distinct regional dialects exist in many countries of Africa and southern Asia. By going away to residential schools in a different area, children are occasionally taught in what is virtually a 'foreign language' and have extreme difficulty in communicating verbally or in writing with their parents and siblings when they return home. 'Local school' attendance enables them to learn their mother tongue as well as to keep abreast of social and family developments - provided, of course, individual tutoring is made available to them. By having the children home each evening, parents and siblings are able to take more interest in them and, with guidance, become more skilled in helping them both educationally and socially.

In 1980, the World Health Organisation divided the world into three groups: the Least Developed Countries (population 283 million); the Developing Countries (3001 million); and the Developed Countries (1131 million). The first two groups thus accounted for almost three-quarters of the world's population. The first group, the Least Developed Countries, was described by Dr Kurt Waldheim as 'the poorest of the poor', and consists of 31 countries:

Africa: Benin, Botswana, Burundi, Cape Verde, Central African Republic, Chad, Comoro Islands, Ethiopia, Gambia, Guinea, Guinea-Bissau, Lesotho, Malawi, Mali, Niger, Rwanda, Somalia, Sudan, Uganda, Tanzania, and Upper Volta.

Asia and Oceania: Afghanistan, Bangladesh, Bhutan, Laos, Maldive Islands, Nepal, People's Democratic Republic of Yemen, Samoa, and Yemen Arab Republic.

Americas: Haiti.

Developing Countries - the Indian experience

A large proportion of the children in the Least Developed and even in the Developing Countries have no schools of any kind to attend, so that integration programmes must be adapted. In India, one of the Developing Countries, Dr N. Rathna and his staff at the All India Institute of Speech and Hearing in Mysore, South India, have had considerable success in remote country districts with week-long 'camps'. (These may have relevance for some of the Least Developed Countries.) Teams of doctors, nurses and speech therapists conduct clinics for the local people. Where an irreversible hearing loss is ascertained,[2] hearing aids are fitted immediately and basic guidance in their use is given to the patient and the village elders. The success rate on revisits has been sufficiently encouraging for the practice to have now become standard. The National individual hearing aids are fitted.*

In Bombay, Poona, Mysore, Delhi, Madras, Calcutta and some other areas of India a number of teachers, audiologists and parents have begun experimental integration programmes. The reports by Mrs Joshi and her teachers in Poona, summarised below, indicate that numerous problems have been encountered, but some of these have been overcome and all teachers and parents could see many positive aspects to educating their children in schools for non-handicapped boys and girls.

Size of ordinary classes and lack of space in ordinary classrooms were often cited as major stumbling blocks to integrating unit classes into ordinary ones.

---

* The British government provides hearing aids free under the National Health Service. Ear-level hearing aids are now fitted to 90 per cent of the children who wear hearing aids in Great Britain. These are slightly more expensive to buy, but the most recent findings are that they are considerably cheaper to maintain. They are also much more easily concealed and, in consequence are worn much more frequently. It may be of significance to Education and Health Departments in some of the Least Developed and Developing Countries that, owing to the large quantities required, these aids can be produced for the British government and other countries at a cost much less than that of similar commercial instruments. The producer is A. and M. Hearing Aids Ltd, Kelvin Way, Crawley, West Sussex, RH10 2LS, England.

Integrating one handicapped child into these classes is much more feasible if support is available.

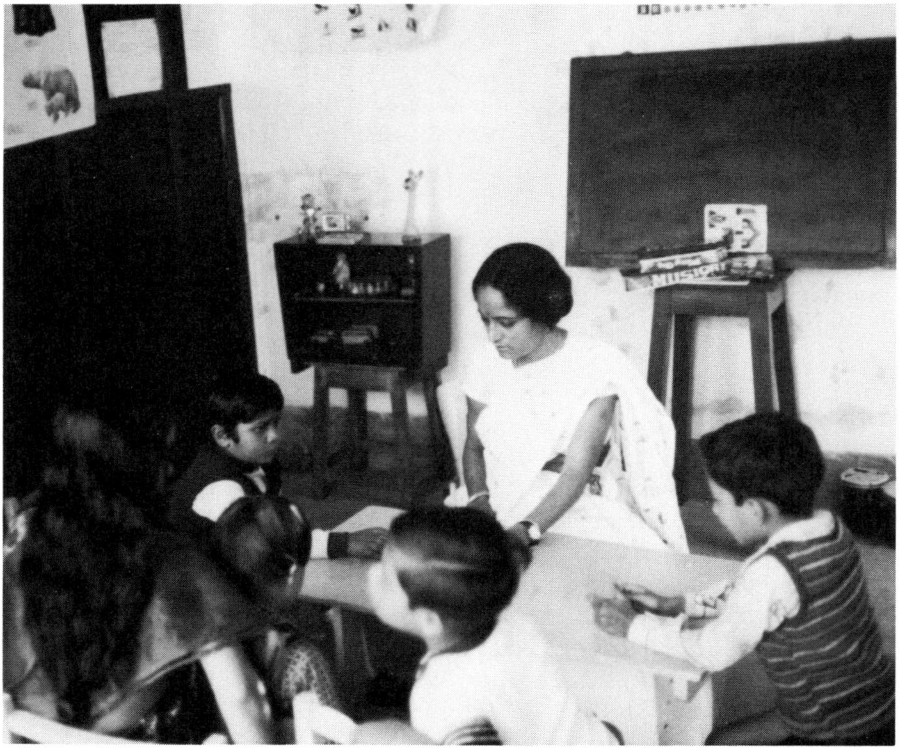

Figure 15 Teaching children in a Calcutta speech and hearing centre before they are transferred to their local ordinary schools, 1981. (A mother can be seen observing.)

Reports of field workers (resource teachers of the deaf) in Poona, India, October 1979

Since 1974, 27 children had been placed in 'good' local ordinary primary and middle schools, or had attended a unit in one of the high schools in the Maharashtra Education Board District of Poona. By 1979, 18 children were so placed in local ordinary classes, as follows:

1st Year	4
2nd Year	1
3rd Year	3
4th Year	2
5th Year	6
7th Year	1
10th Year	1

No accurate details of hearing losses, academic abilities, home potential and so on were available, but all children had previously been admitted to the school for the deaf.

A charitable organisation and Mrs Joshi, the head teacher of V.R. Ruia School for Deaf Children, arranged tutoring by teachers of the deaf for the primary and middle school children at a local centre. The centre was open for two-and-a-half hours each morning from 7.15 a.m., and again from 12.30 to 4.00 p.m. The young children were brought to the centre at pre-arranged times during the morning session and the middle school children for the afternoon session after their ordinary school day had ended. These children usually did their homework from 12.30 to 1.30 p.m.; from 1.30 to 2.30 they had work with the resource teachers; and from 2.30 to 4.00 they did more homework. On Saturday mornings, three hours were spent with the children on revision.

Although both the teachers of the deaf and ordinary school teachers involved were pleased with the scheme so far, the teachers of the deaf did report the following problems (a number of these are, of course, very similar to those encountered in other studies reported in this book).

(1) Distance from the tutoring centre caused problems for parents – particularly those of the younger children.

(2) Most subjects taken in the ordinary classrooms needed to be taught over again and this was time-consuming.

(3) It was difficult to assess how much had been learned in class. In consequence, the resource teachers had found it best to attend the classes with the children whenever they could.

(4) History and abstract language could not be taught exclusively by using pictorial and other visual aids.

(5) Mathematical concepts were also difficult to explain.

(6) Science subjects could be very successful, but usually required modern laboratories and apparatus which were not often available.

(7) Geography needed practical work such as journeys and teaching aids such as slides and good illustrations.

(8) Both the children and the teachers of the deaf sometimes felt overburdened by the amount of work required of them. The children's relaxation and play with friends were often curtailed by the extra hours of work which they were doing. At the secondary (high school) level, similar problems occurred, although since all ten girls were attending the one school, tutoring could be offered (in an art classroom) more easily.

(9) Each week the resource teachers tried to meet the form teachers to discuss the portion of the subject to be covered. Since there were 45 teachers involved with various classes, it was not possible for the two teachers of the deaf to meet all the others each week, and teaching (or tutoring) the various children in a total of about 20 subjects was not at all easy.

In their report, the field workers commented:

> In all these schemes, parents have to play a vital role. For example, they should: work hard to help the child get his/her studies completed each day;

> often make enquiries of the teachers; help the resource teachers; identify where the pupil has interests and encourage him/her to improve upon that subject of interest. If this is done, then pupils have been found to progress. Just sending the child to school is not enough.
>
> India is a poor country. Even basic necessities are difficult. For daily bread, persons are moving to big cities, where they have great problems of accommodation. Under such circumstances, deaf sons or daughters are sometimes treated as a 'curse'. Private charities or the schools for deaf children have often been the parents' mainstays. If parents are educated, they can guide the child well. Much often depended on colleagues, friends and neighbours. All should co-operate – teacher, resource teacher and home. They should share their experiences and thus help each child to make progress.

These excellent teachers were clearly working most assiduously against considerable odds. More itinerant teachers of the deaf and welfare assistants were needed (*see* chapters 5 and 6) but also, some adaptation of the timetables would have helped. Learning additional language dialects and English in the ordinary schools were unnecessarily heavy additional burdens placed upon most deaf children attending ordinary schools in many parts of India, and it was recommended that, for most of them, these additional requirements should be dropped. In a number of regions, this had been approved.

Research Proposal: Individual Integration of Hearing-Impaired Children in Ordinary Schools in Selected Areas in India

The following outline by the writer is included as it is felt that it may have relevance for workers in other developing countries.

Introduction

In 1978, Professor J. Tizard wrote: 'Parliament has decreed that, at some point in the future, all or nearly all children should be educated in ordinary schools. Essentially similar legislation has been passed in the USA, in Italy, France and in Scandinavia, so Section 10 [of the 1976 Education Act[88]] is not just a quirk of a few grey beards in the House of Lords at Westminster.'[223]

Professor Tizard, Research Professor of Child Development (1964–80) at the University of London Institute of Education, went on to point out that not all teachers or parents were yet convinced of the wisdom of 'Section 10'. (This Section has not, in fact, been implemented although the principle is widely accepted.) Chapter 7 of the Warnock Report[232] spelt out the implications of such qualifying conditions as practicability, efficiency and cost if the Section 10 proposal was implemented. For three major reasons, it is suggested that the proposed studies might be implemented in India (and other developing countries).

(1) The alternatives to individualised local ordinary school placement are no

education, units in ordinary schools, or day or residential special schools. The last three of these facilities are very expensive and becoming more so (*see* Table 10, p. 138).
(2) The level of educational achievement and social adjustment achieved in the *majority* of units or special schools for hearing-impaired children in Western countries is disappointing.[46,99,187]
(3) The fact that India and most other Developing Countries have large resources of women who have had a successful primary school education means that they could be employed very effectively on an hourly basis as classroom assistants for each handicapped child. When guided by itinerant specialist teachers and classroom teachers, it is felt that very satisfying results should be possible with most children.

Establishing research groups

The following is the recommended feasibility study (using the Warnock criteria[232] of practicability, efficiency and cost).

Otologists and head teachers of schools for deaf children, working (if possible) with local university or teachers' college staff, should be asked to select up to ten suitable children in collaboration with an overall supervisor. Since the children would be taught in separate schools, they need not be all of one age. Control groups should be selected from the deaf schools. Criteria for the initial selection would be as follows:
(1) Distances between the children's local schools should not be too great. (This saves both the time and the expense of the itinerant teacher, and also makes supervision by senior teachers easier.)
(2) The children should be of at least average intelligence and reasonably well-adjusted socially and emotionally.[190] (Later, the more handicapped children should also certainly be included.)
(3) Some children should be very severely deaf and others partially hearing.
(4) If possible, in this initial programme parents or relatives should be interested in helping the children educationally – or at least be willing to find ways in which they could be helpful.[154]
(5) The local ordinary schools used should also be running at least 'reasonably well', for example, with a sympathetic and efficient head and class teachers.
(6) If class size is large (say 55–60 children) this is a disadvantage, but frequently, if one is able to provide generous support for the deaf child, the scheme could well work to everyone's advantage. For example, the itinerant teacher of the deaf and the supporting classroom assistant often work with the deaf child and two or three other children who the class teacher feels need extra educational help. If the children in the deaf child's remedial group can be from homes near to that of the deaf child, this can be very helpful in establishing friendships for out-of-school hours.
(7) Assessments of each child's educational, social, psychological and audiological capacities should be made.
(8) The itinerant teacher of the deaf should be competent, energetic, tactful and cheerful. She should also be able to drive a car or ride a motor scooter to

enable her to move quickly to see individual children in several schools during each school day.
(9) Monthly reports from each area should be made to the overall research supervisor.
(10) Towards the end of the first school year, assessments of both groups should be made.
(11) There should be a one-week conference of research workers and teachers for a full discussion of results and consideration of modifications found to be necessary. Reports would be sent to medical workers in audiology clinics if they could not attend. If results are generally positive, expansion could be considered not only in the research centres, but also in other areas.

Malawi

The first integration experiment in Malawi was begun at the Montfort Demonstration School in Limbe in October 1980. Three profoundly deaf boys were admitted and a trained teacher of the deaf was appointed to assist them. By March 1982, seven such children had been admitted to this school.

Despite large ordinary class sizes (over 50 children), the class teachers were impressed by these boys' ability to cope with the full breadth of the curriculum. All were deaf as a result of meningitis so they had some language and speech (*see* Table 9).

Table 9 Children admitted to first year preparatory classes in Malawi

Child	Years of age	Aetiology: meningitis	Average hearing loss	Class
1	8	,,	120	2
2	12	,,	100	3
3	13	,,	100	3
4	13	,,	110	5
5	12	,,	100	6
6	12	,,	100	6
7	15	,,	110	8

The teacher of the deaf was delighted with the warm reception given to these profoundly deaf children by both the teachers and their classmates. Each deaf child was allocated a bright, normally hearing child to act as a friend who could be asked by the teacher to help him and generally keep him informed of what was happening in the class. The teacher of the deaf reported that this assistance was not necessary 'all the time' – and that it had worked well. Comments from the ordinary school teachers since this experiment began have been very favourable, for example, 'I never knew that a deaf child could be taught successfully in a normal school.'

The aim in this initial experiment was that, when a deaf child was successful, he should be transferred to his local school for normally hearing children.

Thereafter, it was intended to follow them up with visits and to receive written reports from class teachers.

This writer has suggested that rather more daily coaching assistance from itinerant teachers and/or from intelligent people living locally would be necessary for most of these profoundly deaf children if they were to derive maximum benefit from these placements. (*See* chapters 6 and 8.)

8

Post-school education

During the 1960s, colleges of further education in the United States began admitting increasing numbers of hearing-impaired students – both in groups and individually.[37,143,214] Teachers of the deaf, social workers and interpreters were employed to help these students derive maximum benefit from a wide variety of courses (Appendix 7, page 195). In the United Kingdom, too, the Russell Report on Adult Education made repeated recommendations that 'adults who are handicapped or disadvantaged in others ways, should be given special consideration'.[193] By the late 1960s and early 1970s, serious attempts were being made in the United Kingdom to provide full- and part-time courses and evening classes for young hearing-impaired adults, and in 1974–5 over 200 post-school courses were available at United Kingdom colleges (*see* Appendix 8, pages 196–9). It is considered that any of these might prove of interest to deaf or partially hearing students, provided that supporting services were made available.

A survey of 20 institutions of further education in England

A brief survey of 20 institutions offering tertiary education in the north and south of England was conducted by F.W. Slade and the writer in 1974–5, using structured interviews (*see* Appendix 9, pages 200–1). Eleven of these colleges had not previously admitted deaf students, and the remaining nine had had between three and seven years' experience in this field.

The 11 colleges reacted very positively to the enquiry as to whether they would consider admitting hearing-impaired students at some future time, and indeed it was encouraging that a great deal of goodwill was seen to exist among these heads of colleges. In fact, provided that consideration was given to supporting the deaf students, *all* the institutions surveyed were pleased to admit them.

A more detailed study was made in the nine colleges where a number of severely handicapped students had already been enrolled. These colleges were:

The City Literary Institute, London
The Brixton College, London
The Royal School for the Deaf, Derby
Finchale Training College, near Durham
Tewin Water Further Education Department, Hertfordshire
Derwent Training College and Workshop for the Disabled, Oswestry, Shropshire
Bournville College of Further Education, Birmingham
Hereward College of Further Education for the Physically Handicapped, Coventry
Shirecliffe College, Sheffield

Thirty-six members of staff interviewed at these colleges considered that the development and expansion of suitable courses for handicapped students were both possible and desirable. In one instance, however, four lecturers felt that 'saturation point' had about been reached, owing to economic, social and other factors.

Most lecturers felt that the greatest problem for the deaf student was language deprivation, and that it was most desirable to concentrate on the use of language (basic and technical) both before students enrolled on courses and after the courses had begun.

Points made by staff during their interviews

Preliminary considerations

* A separate file should be kept on each student.
* 'Link courses' between the deaf schools and the colleges were very popular and enabled the deaf student to obtain a clear picture of the possibilities and the problems to be encountered when he or she attended full-time the following year (*see* Appendix 10, pp. 201–2).
* Parental interest was of great importance. At Sheffield, parents were asked to attend an evening meeting one week before the first term began where it was stressed to them that follow-up of work by parents (or siblings) could be *vital*. Some parents had to be helped to realise this and be given careful guidance in the ways in which they could show their interest and offer assistance.
* The extra time that the new course was going to demand had to be discussed. Students (and parents) had to realise that things were not going to be easy – 'there should be no illusions about this'. With the right attitude, however, things would go well and, in fact, the students observed certainly appeared to be enjoying this new responsibility and challenge.
* All students (in two areas) were given the home telephone number of their tutor-teacher of the deaf. A member of their family could then telephone if they had problems that needed resolving urgently.

* In larger colleges, teachers of the deaf were quite adamant that, if a member of the college staff seemed diffident or indifferent at the outset, they would quickly find someone else who seemed more responsive. In the smaller colleges, of course, such choice of lecturer was often not available.
* One tutor commented: 'Our deaf youngsters are very much in the minority so we can't expect the college to adapt a whole course for the sake of one student.' Other tutors, however, had noted that, among the normally hearing students, there was a large group incapable of dealing adequately with certain aspects of college work such as examinations, lectures, textbooks and timetables. That is, there is low performance among a number of normally hearing students and this is a great help to any slow or poorly educated deaf students.
* During preliminary visits, students were advised to 'keep an open mind about courses and to look at as many courses as possible'.
* Group and individual meetings with specialists and parents to discuss the most appropriate course were considered to be most successful.
* 'Avoid classes for deaf students only.' This comment was frequently made by lecturers in Sheffield, Derby and London.
* One college in Sheffield and one in London said that, so far, they had been able to accept every student who had applied to come on a further education course.
* The deputy head of one college said: 'We are all in favour of integration, provided effective support services are available – money, staff and facilities. We sometimes recommend one course rather than another because staff are more sympathetic. Some staff have even helped students with their transport to college – offering lifts in their cars and so on.'

The first weeks

* 'The lecturers have been excellent but they do need a great deal of help from teachers of the deaf.'
* It had been found valuable to talk early in the year to the normally hearing students in the class about the problem of communication for the deaf student. They wanted to help the handicapped students but didn't know where to begin.
* Lipreading classes for the deaf students should be offered. These are also found in the Rochester Technical Institute for the Deaf programme (pp. 52–3). Video-tape cassettes can be made containing common words in short phrases spoken by the lecturer in a particular subject.
* Lipreading a speaker who was not using his voice helped normally hearing students understand some of the problems of their deaf colleagues.

During the course

In Derby, three wine and cheese parties were held by the lecturers in deaf education and the deaf students at the deaf school or the further education residential unit. These were at the beginning and end of the academic year and at Christmas time. They were for the staff of the colleges who were involved. The students enjoyed acting as hosts and hostesses. These gatherings were felt to be a tangible way of saying thank-you to those engaged in the work and also afforded an opportunity for the lecturers to compare methods of presenting information to their respective students.

Initially, the deaf students were much slower than the normally hearing ones at reading and answering examination questions. Some tutor teachers of the deaf obtained an extension of time for some of their students; others helped rewrite questions so that they would be more intelligible to the deaf students and, it was often observed by the lecturers, more intelligible to the normally hearing students also. (If examinations are adapted too much, however, they are not of equal difficulty and the deaf student then obtains a qualification which is not comparable to that obtained by his or her normally hearing counterparts.) The theory aspects of courses were always difficult but it was a great help if the technical language could be mastered.

Socially, the students at Derby 'got on well with the hearing students in class each day, but tended to congregate with the other deaf students who stayed at their hostel in the evenings'. (The warden and his wife asked to know where the students were going in the evenings and what time they would be coming home. 'It all works very well,' they said.)

The staff at one college made the following negative points which, although real enough, can often be overcome by initial training for all concerned and continuing care and attention when the programme is running:

* 'The deaf are reluctant to seek help.'
* 'Some students play on their deafness.'
* 'Lecturers say, "You have got a new hearing aid so now you can hear."'
* 'Mature students [with 50 dB hearing losses] think they can hear everything.'
* 'The deaf have frustrations of placement in further education.'

Three times a year, non-academic reports were made on students at one college. Students saw these reports, which could be modified before they were finally typed.

Other points raised by staff included:

* 'I do a great deal of work with parents and the careers service have been enormously helpful' (London advisory tutor of deaf students).
* Ordinary college lecturers said they had found 'a tremendous desire for knowledge' among many of the deaf students which they had not previously encountered in either 'normal' students, or those with other handicaps.
* Attending the London colleges individually had 'built up the confidence of deaf students enormously'.
* In Sheffield, Derby and, recently, in London, students who progressed best socially, and often academically, were those who went singly to classes. If there were two deaf students, the normally hearing students were disinclined to become involved with them. This has been noted in other studies.[56]
* According to one tutor in London, some of the deaf students used the

City Literary Institute as a social centre – 'Just for an hour or so, once or twice a month. They need to unwind.' This excellent tutor had previously spent five years as a principal of a teachers' college in Africa and recalled that, in those days, although enjoying her work enormously, she would sometimes travel 30 miles to spend just one hour with some English people – 'not American or Swedish or Australian – but *English*!' (This point should be borne in mind by all who are integrating severely handicapped people individually into schools and colleges.)

Ordinary college lecturers interviewed in Sheffield, Derby and London felt that ample preparation and use of visual aids, including written handouts and blackboard summaries, helped communicate information a great deal, and lipreading plus a few basic gestures seemed to get most information across very effectively. They were quite strongly against the use of manual methods and felt that a number of students had improved markedly since leaving the deaf schools and having to rely on the above methods.

Tape recorders were found useful for certain students. Partially hearing students could listen to these, and severely deaf ones had tapes typed for parts of courses. Typing of the taped material could be a problem, but some students would offer to do this and occasionally an office secretary when she had time. If six or seven lectures a day were taped, however, the amount of reading involved for the student was found to be too great. Deaf students occasionally borrowed a competent student's notes, the deaf student typing up the material and giving a copy to the normally hearing student – similar to Dr James Marsters' technique reported below (p. 118). A third method, occasionally used was that of obtaining a copy of the previous year's notebook from a competent, normally hearing student. The deaf student could then read the lecture before, during and after the teaching session.

Regular written work throughout the year was considered to be quite essential.

Problems and successes during the course were discussed each week at individual tutorials with each student, as well as giving the students an opportunity to consider any social aspects that they felt were causing concern. At one college, deaf students were counselled once each term when their parents were present.

Further education for individual deaf students in Sheffield

Excellent work has been carried out in Sheffield since 1968, largely through the efforts of the lecturers in education of the deaf and their colleagues on the staffs of the four colleges of further education. The staff of the school for deaf children also collaborated fully in this development. The following notes are adapted from a report by the senior lecturer in the education of deaf students, and are felt to be useful both to other teachers/lecturers in charge of deaf students and to college lecturers who are about to teach a deaf student.

The policy of teaching the hearing-impaired student in further education in Sheffield is one of integration wherever possible, supported by *individual* teaching. Each student has individual teaching in English and communication from a qualified teacher of the deaf, but also the aim is to provide *individual* tutorials with technical teachers (Appendix 11, pp. 202–3).

Although the technical teachers are not qualified teachers of the deaf, the enthusiasm and interest they have for their subject is felt to provide a more useful teaching situation than would a teacher of the deaf working from technical notes. These tutors have had instruction on methods of teaching the deaf and on communication from the further education teacher of the deaf. They also have advice and help in the classroom and an opportunity to watch the teacher of the deaf at work in the classroom. Very close co-operation and teamwork is required from all concerned.

At an inter-college meeting of tutors of deaf students, the following points were discussed:

Tutorials – individual teaching from a teacher of the technical subject.
There are several benefits:

- ★ The deaf student has an opportunity to work on points he may not have understood in the classroom and has some extra teaching.
- ★ Extra time need not be spent in the classroom on the single deaf student (which could be to the detriment of the other students), because their difficulties could be dealt with at their tutorials.
- ★ The deaf student has the opportunity of getting to know one member of staff better, so possibly will think of this person as a friend and can refer to him or her for other difficulties in college.

It was emphasised by all individuals concerned that the tutorials with deaf students were very demanding mentally and also in terms of both work preparation and re-orientation.

It was felt strongly that each tutor must care for the deaf student as a human being first and foremost. The handicap was responsible for the mode of approach, but the student was primarily a *person* who happened to be deaf. If anyone took on the tutorial teaching for other motives, or as just a job that had to be done, he or she could expect failure.

Teaching aids

There should be some re-thinking about the way material is presented by lecturers who have deaf students in the classroom. There must be a bias towards visual aids:

- ★ More use of the blackboard.
- ★ More use of the overhead projector.
- ★ More use of handouts.
- ★ The possibility of carbon copies of lecture notes from other able students.
- ★ Laboratory work and practical work to be allied to the theoretical work where possible.

It was suggested by one lecturer that because he had rethought his methods of presentation to help the one deaf student, this simplified, clearer approach had obviously helped the rest of the group as was shown by the higher level of examination results.

Problems of the deaf student

The chief problem, repeated again and again, was the lack of language and the lack of understanding of language on the part of the deaf student. No one was unduly concerned by problems of communication.

The tutor must make sure that the deaf student really understands the subject matter and is not just appearing to understand. The student must be constantly encouraged to ask questions when necessary. Sometimes, he/she may not ask for help because of a desire to show independence and an unwillingness to admit difficulties. Some deaf students also appeared to over-estimate their ability and their performance in examinations.

Personal problems could affect their performance in college. Deaf boys tended to have difficulty with girlfriends. Deaf girls preferred to marry hearing men if possible, and hearing girls were sometimes disinclined to associate with deaf boys because of the speech and language difficulties.

A deaf student, like a normally hearing one, could be lacking in motivation and co-operation. It was naïve to imagine that all deaf students were otherwise. The lecturer must be careful that allowances for the handicap did not take up too much of his teaching. For a handicapped student to succeed, he or she must be well motivated and prepared to work harder than most other students.

Attitudes of schools

Schools should pass on to the college complete information about a student and be completely honest. Lecturers felt that there was more to teaching deaf students than the imparting of technical information. They needed to know something about previous behaviour problems and home background as all this could influence the student's performance in college.

There had been several cases where the student had been totally disinterested in the craft part of the course. Ability with the hands is a vital requirement for a deaf student, and if this is lacking, there is no point in lecturers struggling with the theory work. It is therefore essential that schools make sure, from work experiences and careers guidance, that the pupil is appropriately placed.

Further useful points were made by Jean Sutton, the senior teacher of the deaf, during a lecture in 1980.[216] According to Mrs Sutton, some of the students who were top of their class in the deaf school were bottom of the class at the ordinary college. This could be demoralising, and at such times they would be told of other students who had had similar early experiences and yet succeeded after a year or two. Sometimes these same students had come top of the ordinary class by the end of the third or fourth year.

It was explained to the deaf students that normally hearing students had three pathways to help them learn: the visual, kinaesthetic and the auditory. Without perfect hearing, the deaf students found it harder to learn and, in consequence, it was necessary to work really hard to achieve near normal results. It is not always easy for a young person to accept this, but the staff pointed out that the course of two, three or four years, although seeming a long time, was, in fact, a short period of one's working life and therefore it was well worthwhile to make the effort.

Reading material on terminology was given to the deaf students and each was able to build up a personal dictionary.

Although the lecturers in the various subjects used speech, writing and a few gestures, in her individual tutoring sessions the senior teacher of the deaf, Jean Sutton, said she used a mixture of talking, writing, signing, finger spelling and gestures – 'anything that keeps the interchange of ideas flowing'.

Lecturers' example was important – not just in the way they groomed and dressed themselves, but also in their punctuality, their loyalty to one another, their preparation of work and their general attitude to their work. One way of helping the young deaf students with their problems was for lecturers to discuss some of their own problems. For example, they talked about how they were going about selecting their next car – whether to buy a new or a second-hand one; when the college closed during a caretakers' strike, the pros and cons of striking were discussed; if they were feeling sad one day, they might talk about the reasons. Current events were useful topics for discussion and newspapers were important for this.[56]

Once a year an 'open evening' was held at the base college. Pupils from the deaf school who were within 18 months of leaving school were invited as were their parents; lecturers from all the colleges concerned with courses taken by deaf students and also some of the present students and their parents came. The senior teacher of the deaf gave a general talk and then students proudly conducted the visitors around the college. Worried parents of future students could discuss their concerns with the other parents and staff members present. The lecturers from the other colleges were there to discuss the courses in which they were engaged, and visits to the other colleges were arranged as required. These evenings have been considered to be thoroughly worthwhile by all concerned.

Deaf people's suggestions

Ex-students of a splendid school for deaf children in the United States – Clarke School in Northampton, Massachusetts – made the following suggestions to children who were about to leave the school. Virtually all of these practical points can be related directly to a deaf person's integration into ordinary society.

- ★ Do as many things as possible with hearing people.
- ★ Learn how to ask questions.
- ★ Take part in as many activities as possible.
- ★ Don't expect any special favours because you are deaf.
- ★ Learn how to feel at home with hearing people. Practise it.

- ★ Learn how to make friends. Don't wait for the hearing people to come to you.
- ★ Put the hearing people at ease by being at ease yourself.
- ★ Always be well-dressed and well-mannered.
- ★ Learn to live with both the hearing and the deaf and enjoy both.
- ★ Try not to work next to another deaf person. You'll work better and get along better with the hearing people if you are on your own.
- ★ Explain your handicap at certain times. It will educate the public.
- ★ Don't become discouraged too easily. Remember, others have passed through the same situations and were less well-prepared.
- ★ Get all of the educational and vocational training possible.
- ★ Try to keep up with current 'slang' and what is popular.
- ★ Don't limit your associates to a small group. Deaf clubs should be a small part of your social life.
- ★ Read, read, read.

Observations by profoundly deaf adults who have received tertiary education in ordinary colleges or universities are particularly valuable. Practical guidance and encouragement can be given to other deaf students and their parents and to the professionals engaged in this work. It can be seen, for example, that most of the problems which Dr Marsters describes below (and which Mrs Dolbear has described in chapter 3) could have been prevented by even a little intervention by an experienced teacher of the deaf or a sensitive lecturer. Support is also necessary outside the college, and it is heartening to notice that both Mrs Dolbear and Dr Marsters have acknowledged the debt they owe to their parents.

It is not suggested that *all* deaf people could achieve as much as Dr Marsters and the other brilliant people described in chapter 3. Indeed, the majority would certainly not. With adequate support, however, a large proportion of young deaf people are able to cope educationally and socially in ordinary colleges and universities.

Dr James C. Marsters, DDS

The following is an account of the university education and professional life of Dr James C. Marsters, who has been profoundly deaf from birth.

> I matriculated at Union College, Schenectady, NY, in 1943. I chose to go there so that I would feel a part of a small college, rather than being lost in a large university. I am glad I chose this route, as I became a fencing coach, writer and manager of the college newspaper and a member of Sigma Chi fraternity, and was involved in a multitude of other activities in addition to my academic work. I also washed dishes, waited tables, did garden work and put on magic shows to help pay my way through college. I felt that it was important for me to learn to survive and compete well with my hearing peers on *their* terms, as this was the way things worked in the outside world.

The only tutoring I had was for German, as the professor wanted me to learn to speak it; I agreed (realizing that the professor was not being very realistic), and he soon learned it was better for me to learn written and printed German. There were no special considerations for me in college – no interpreters, or paid note-takers, as deaf students so usefully receive today from state or federal grants. I would copy the notes of my classmates on either side of me, or in front of me ... or just read them if things were moving too fast – borrowing those of the best note-takers and typing them up and giving them a copy. Researching in the library was necessary as well, of course.

Most important was studying the course materials before attending the classes so I would have a good picture of what was going to be presented and hence a better understanding during the repeat. I could not borrow the professor's notes, as most of them did not have good ones, but things are often better today in the larger universities where some professors have their lectures typed for handouts or printed for publication and so on.

There were times when I was very angry about being in a classroom and not being able to 'take it easy' like my classmates, and about being 'wiped out' by being deprived of auditory learning and class discussions. A few times I would leave the classrooms because of my frustration. Although there was great temptation to stay out and study in the library or in my room, I was aware that once I started doing this I would no longer be a part of the class and the student body, and so would defeat myself by segregating myself... so I continued attending classes.

A geology professor did not want me in his classroom, as he did not wish 'to be responsible' for me. I went to him and said that I did not want him to be responsible for me either; I would take care of myself, but would appreciate a consultation after classes once in a while regarding important materials to be covered. He finally agreed and later, as classes progressed, asked me to major in geology. I majored in pre-medicine and psychology. I had to take required courses not only in my majors, but also in liberal arts subjects. I graduated with my classmates, and stayed on for another semester.

While an undergraduate, I married an oral deaf girl. I wanted to be a psychiatrist and so I applied to Syracuse University Medical School but was not accepted. I felt I would probably not make a good physician, as I would not be able to encourage good communication, which is so essential in medical practice. (I feel now, however, that I was wrong then, and that it would have been quite possible. Today, we have two or three profoundly deaf physicians in the USA.)

My wife and I moved to New York City, where I tried, with degree in hand, to find jobs in chemistry and many other fields, being turned down, I think, because I was deaf and also lacked sufficient work experience in the fields. This was a very sobering and upsetting experience. I finally found work in a necktie fabric firm but did not enjoy it. One day the boss asked me 'out of the blue' why I should not consider dentistry. I reacted saying I did not like dentists. He then asked if I enjoyed using my hands, since I had been a professional magician. I said yes. He said, well that's dentistry, too. Also, he said, I seemed to enjoy helping people, as he had seen me helping a number of my workmates. In addition to this I could be my own boss and live where I wanted to. 'So, why not take the afternoon off and visit the dental school?' This I did. From then on I was 'hooked' on dentistry. The ugly experience of being under-employed and under-challenged had proved both depriving and demeaning.

Applications to five dental schools met with rejections from four. One, New York University, sent me in for 40 hours of aptitude testing along with other qualified applicants – 1400 for 150 positions. (Many were already graduate students trying to avoid being drafted in the Korean War.) The Board of Admissions interviewed me ... and each professor asked me why I didn't go into his field, instead of being a dentist ... having just found that I was profoundly deaf. I explained to them that I preferred working with and helping people to being sequestered in a laboratory. The dean summed up things: 'Mr Marsters, in all of my 35 years of teaching dentistry, I have never heard of a deaf dental student.' I replied cheerily: 'Fine! Why don't you give it a try?' I was rejected. For the next year I encouraged the professors at the NY Dental School to 'give it a try' and they finally obliged by letting me in on probation. (I had spent some time taking dental technician courses beforehand to improve my skills while trying to get into dental school.)

Medical and dental schools were very demanding, but I found that I could help classmates where they were weak and I was strong, and vice versa. It was very difficult doing the course work, as professors are often difficult to lipread, being bored with their own repetitious lecturing. As before, I would find the best note-takers and ask if they would like me to type up their notes for them and return them the next day ... in other words, helping them as well as myself. Learning to cope and to survive was the name of the game, and prior bitter experiences of being denied a rewarding job or position drove me on, determined to succeed. Again, I had no interpreters or paid note-takers. (Today, my nurses help by interpreting orally for me when I am using the voice telephone – telling me what the other party is saying while they say it and then I do my own thinking and talking on the telephone – or, if a patient is extremely difficult to lipread, I will ask my nurse to oral interpret for me.)

I graduated with my class with a degree of Doctor of Dental Surgery in the standard four years and took licenses both in the states of New York and California, the latter having the reputation of being the most difficult to secure, but then, I always wanted to live in California ... I opened a general practice of dentistry in Pasadena, California, and this continued for two years. I also attended the University of Southern California graduate school to become a specialist in orthodontics – straightening the teeth of adults as well as children so they may have healthier and stronger teeth

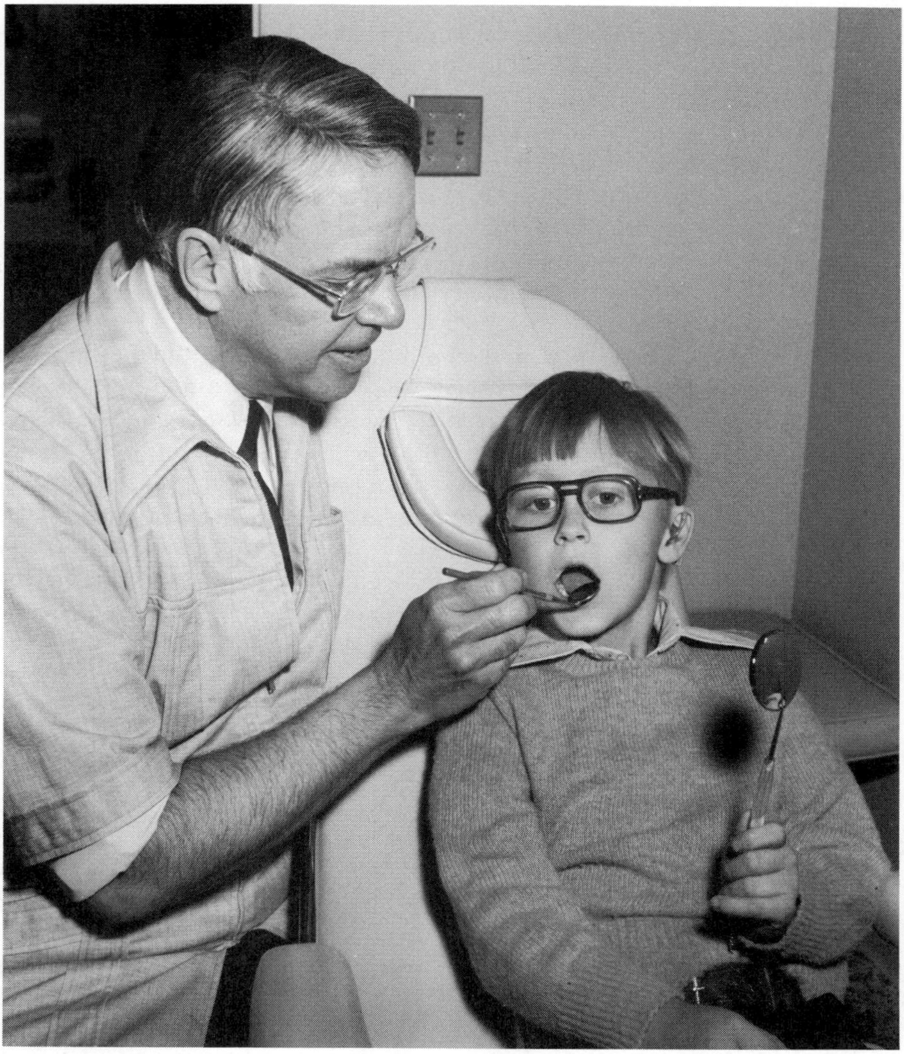

Figure 16 Dr James Marsters, profoundly deaf from birth, examines a patient.

over a lifetime as well as being more beautiful. At times this also involves maxialla-facial surgery. I enjoy the general practice of dentistry, working with all kinds of people and all kinds of dental work, but I have preferred the challenge of orthodontics.

In 1954 I was awarded a Master of Science degree and proceeded to open an orthodontic speciality practice in Pasadena. I also continued to teach in the undergraduate and graduate schools at the University of Southern California, lecturing and clinical demonstrations. My practice in a few years grew to a point where I had to discontinue teaching and devote full time to it. I also opened a second office in Lone Pine, California. I fly my airplane back and forth to it for which I have had a pilot's license for a long time. (A waiver was secured for my deafness as I fly alone most of the time. I also like to soar gliders.)

I have now practised orthodontics for 25 years and enjoy it very much. There are continual challenges every day to do better, as the competition is very strong, as well as the care of different kinds of patients. Less than one percent of my practice involves hearing-impaired people, so I must continue to improve my skills in interpersonal communication with the hearing world (as well as with myself). Improvements in speech and voice were also sought.

While in college and dental schools I wore a hearing aid, as this seemed to make people feel that I was hard of hearing rather than deaf, and I would abet this feeling. Today, I no longer wear a hearing aid, as it seems of minimal benefit and I do not need it. It is rare that a patient will decline to come to me due to my deafness. I am very sensitive to their feelings and fears, and know when I am hurting them. I give them a way to control me when they wish.

I am very keen that deaf babies and young children should be fitted with hearing aids and trained in auditory training, as well as in all the other very necessary interpersonal communicative skills and developments. It is all too easy to maintain the status quo, but very scary to maintain continual personal growth, in addition to academic growth, which is so essential to our survival in this highly competitive world. Today the professional fields are opening up still more, as we have more deaf dentists, physicians, architects, accountants and so on who are very capable.

In 1955 I married Alice Dorsey, Director of the John Tracy Clinic Nursery School. (I had lost my deaf wife while attending dental school which took so much of my time.) Alice and I have three hearing children.

The fact that my parents and teachers continued to give me love, encouragement and opportunities, and believed in me from early childhood is the most important factor in my success and survival today.

One can secure a degree in a field, and licenses to practice, but it also takes a lot more to become and remain successful: one has to market one's skills to the public continually. It is important to help people forget I am deaf, as then I overcome my second biggest handicap/block. The *first* biggest handicap is having the wrong attitude.

Educating hearing-impaired students individually in ordinary colleges is currently receiving increasing attention in many Western countries.[212,214,216] It represents one of the most exciting developments in the field – due, in part, to the excellent facilities that have been developed in modern colleges of technology and further education; to the interest of both the professional and practical abilities of many of the staff; to the encouragement and stimulation which has been given to the teachers of the deaf who support these students; and, not least, to the ability of the deaf and normally hearing students to become introspective and make positive criticisms and suggestions for the improvement of the deaf students' opportunities to learn. Recommendations for further education programmes are included in the final chapter of this book.

PART III

Administrative considerations and recommendations

9

Staffing requirements and duties

Co-ordinators

The Warnock Report on Children with Special Needs (1978)[232] recommended that as soon as a child was identified as being in need of special care' 'a named person' should be appointed to act as 'key worker' or 'co-ordinator'. This person was to act as a friend to the family, and was to be entrusted with the task of ensuring that any recommendations made regarding the child were carried out and that all the relevant services and facilities were mobilised. Unfortunately, the Education Act of 1981 did not recommend the appointment of the 'named person'. No doubt, however, public health nurses, advisory teachers of the deaf and head teachers will continue to act in this capacity, but without the title.

Health visitors – in other words, trained nurses who have had additional training in the fields of public and school health nursing – are often particularly well-qualified to help parents during the first years of the handicapped child's life, when many of the parents' queries are concerned with problems of all babies and are not necessarily only those relating to the child's handicap. As children grow older, however, it has been found that teachers who have had training relating to the child's major handicap, and also training in pre-school work, can be extremely helpful to parents. If they have had children of their own, of course, so much the better, since they can often be more practical and realistic in what they ask parents to do in the home training of their deaf children. In a growing number of areas, health visitors and peripatetic teachers of the deaf have collaborated very well in dealing with such children and every encouragement should be given to them to do so through joint meetings during initial and in-service training programmes, attending lectures of mutual interest and holding informal but regular meetings to discuss specific problems.

The Warnock Report states: 'parents can be effective partners only if professionals take notice of what they say and of how they express their needs and treat their contributions as intrinsically important.' This report may, itself, be criticised, however, for not emphasising the importance of identifying, at pre-school level, the large group of children with less severe special needs (perhaps one in six) and recommending early intervention to help them.

At school age, the professional person who assists each family with a handicapped child is often the head teacher of the child's school. Concern has been expressed about this when the head teacher is not available during school holidays, but some arrangements can frequently be made with health visitors during such periods. Some advisory teachers have rearranged their programmes – taking days off during the term – so that parent-guidance visits can be made more regularly during holidays.

The Warnock Report, in chapter 4, wisely recommends that 'education for parenthood' should be offered to all children before they leave school. This would help ensure that future mothers would receive appropriate ante-natal and post-natal care as well as both future mothers and fathers obtaining a clearer picture of what parenthood entails.

Advisory teachers of the deaf

These are sometimes called 'peripatetic'*, 'itinerant', 'travelling' or 'specialist visiting' teachers of the deaf. In this book, however, 'itinerant teachers of the deaf' refer to those who restrict themselves to offering individual assistance to hearing-impaired children in ordinary schools, and to the parents and teachers of these children.

Advisory teachers are usually, but not always, recruited from *experienced* members of the staffs of deaf schools and units. A number of advisory teachers have taken Diplomas in Audiology. In the United Kingdom since 1973, a number have also attended short additional training courses at the universities of Manchester and London. According to a Department of Education and Science Survey in 1969:

> The central function of the advisory service as it has developed and as agreed by the teachers, appears to be guidance for parents of young children and for teachers in ordinary schools.[75]

An indication of the popularity of this service is that, whereas there were four advisory teachers of the deaf in the United Kingdom in 1958, by 1983, over 500 were employed. Each has an area of an education authority or school district for which he or she is responsible, although occasionally one teacher will specialise in work with young children and another with the elder group. This, of course, can double the amount of mileage covered, but it clearly has advantages in certain cases.

The various duties of advisory teachers are described below.

---

* This is defined in the *Concise Oxford Dictionary* as: 1. Aristotelian [from Aristotle's custom of walking in Lyceum while teaching]. 2. Walking from place to place on one's business.

Guidance to parents of pre-school children

When parents are well-informed and encouraged, it has been found that many children who would otherwise grow up wordless can begin to comprehend and use speech before entering school. Their training in all other aspects of living is then much easier as well as their individual integration into ordinary schools and society.

The following procedure is often adopted. As accurate an assessment as possible of the child's hearing loss is obtained. The medical officer of health is informed and an otological report is obtained if the child has not already been referred from these sources.[3]

The home is visited by the advisory teacher at the earliest opportunity after a severe hearing loss has been confirmed – preferably at a time when both parents are present. On this visit the teacher might: note whether the parents are reasonably well-adjusted to the child's handicap; gauge the potential of the home from the point of view of home-training of the child; demonstration how to talk to, and work with, the child; discuss the importance but also the limitations of hearing aids; in certain cases suggest that the parents enroll with the John Tracy Clinic Correspondence Course, 806 West Adams Boulevard, Los Angeles, CA 90007; leave pertinent printed material and begin to keep a personal guidance file, noting requests and comments from parents and what suggestions were made to them. Parents need time to adjust to learning that their child has a serious handicap and teachers must be sensitive to this.

A psychological report is obtained from the educational psychologist responsible for the child's area, as soon as possible. This report will provide information about intellectual and emotional factors and about aspects of the home environment. (Ideally, each hearing-impaired child should be seen routinely by an educational psychologist at least three times during his or her early career – for example, pre-school, at, say, six years and again at 11 years. Some children, of course, with special needs, are seen much more frequently.)

The case is reported by the advisory teacher to the supervising authority in a monthly report.

Home-assistant support can be arranged when there are particular difficulties in a home and often just to give all parents of young deaf children additional support and encouragement.

Guidance to kindergarten teachers and play-centre supervisors

When a deaf child is enrolled at a kindergarten or play centre the teacher in charge is regarded as a 'substitute' mother and given similar guidance. One-day introductory courses of training conducted at the deaf school or some other centre can be invaluable for these teachers and their assistants (*see* chapter 6).

Assistance to children with defective hearing in ordinary schools

Only children with average hearing losses in excess of 25 decibels (dB) in the better ear are the concern of advisory teachers of the deaf. It is well-known that slight deafness, often of the conductive (middle ear) type, can be common. Although, as Owrid and Hamilton[170] have shown, such slight losses can cause educational retardation, their audiological problem does not warrant the use of specialist teachers of the deaf; in other words, remedial teachers can manage them very effectively. Notes for remedial and class teachers are included later in this chapter.

The handicap is assessed (*see* chapter 10) with special reference to:

★ Degree of hearing loss: pure tone and speech tests of hearing and impedance measurements are administered – if possible when parents are present.
★ Educational attainment: reading, arithmetic and speech ability are tested. Further relevant information is obtained from the head teacher and/or class teacher and from any of the child's earlier progress and achievement records.
★ Academic attainment: results of any standardised tests are noted and the teachers' rating of the child's academic ability is also obtained.
★ Any other handicaps, physical or environmental, are noted.
★ An assessment of the child's social adjustment is made.

Appropriate guidance is given to those concerned with the deaf child. Visiting teachers help teachers and pupils to accept the deaf child by explaining some of his interests and abilities, and by demonstrating how to speak to him and involve him in activities. The home is visited if the case seems a sufficiently serious one, and in certain cases, selected sections of a correspondence course are arranged (*see* Appendix 12, pp. 203–8). The referee and medical officer of health for the area are notified, and the case is reported to the teacher's supervising authority.

Assisting children from schools for the deaf and units who transfer to local ordinary schools and colleges

Children who have spent all or most of their earlier school life in a school for the deaf are quite frequently transferred to their local primary or secondary schools or colleges of further education. It is a function of some advisory teachers to help schools prepare the way for these transfers by providing the receiving school or college with information and advice about the child and his likely problems and needs, to enable staff and pupils to make the most suitable arrangements for the deaf pupil. An *itinerant teacher of the deaf* or a *support teacher* visits such children from one to five times each week depending on each child's disability. Regular visits are also made by advisory teachers while the children remain in the school and, where possible, the teachers can undertake regular teaching sessions of severely handicapped children.

Correspondence school lessons★ (now called 'distance teaching') in the

★ See page 90.

verbal subjects have been arranged for some of these children in some countries.[33,97,102,168]

Assistance to employers

It can be an important function of the advisory teacher and, of course, careers officers and social workers, to help deaf school leavers to adjust to working conditions and assist employers and fellow workers to understand and communicate with them. It is usually easier for an 'outsider' to discuss a child's abilities and limitations with employers than it is for parents – although, of course, parents do usually maintain a real interest in the child's welfare when he starts work and after.

Although frequently becoming involved in a limited but very important advisory and supervisory role, advisory teachers are usually not able to help a great deal with the vocational placement and general care of those adult deaf people who require it after they leave school. My own experience suggests that there seems to be a 'hard core' of deaf people (about two or three per cent, for example) who have a great deal of difficulty obtaining and retaining satisfactory employment.

Finding work and accommodation for this group can be time-consuming, and it now seems more generally accepted that welfare officers who have had additional training are a necessity for some deaf adults.[47] As well as the small group mentioned above, there are, of course, the elderly and infirm deaf people who are not always able to be assisted sufficiently by their families or friends. It should also be mentioned, however, that, as with deaf children in ordinary schools, there is a danger of *oversupporting* adults and this can be counterproductive.

Information services

Additional functions of advisory teachers have included:

* Assisting school libraries through school library services to acquire books on handicapped children – for both children and teachers.
* Informing teachers and parents about relevant courses, events and conferences (for example, *see* Appendixes 13 and 14, pp. 209–12).
* Reviewing articles in certain educational journals and making available to teachers information on current developments in the education of children with special needs.

Wherever possible, advisory teachers take opportunities to give information about the special problems of deaf children and adults and to enlist public support in projects for their welfare. The smaller Rotary Clubs, church and women's groups, Red Cross organisations and so on usually appreciate talks – especially when tape recordings of filtered speech and the speech of children are used as well as slides.

Itinerant teachers of the deaf

A recent innovation in many countries has been the development of the itinerant specialist who controls and facilitates support services for handicapped children in ordinary schools. These teachers have been variously called itinerant teachers, support teachers, consultants for hearing services or integration specialists. Their functions vary considerably in different areas, and a number have been outlined in chapters 5 and 6.

In the San Diego School District, California, the itinerant teacher programme began in 1974 with one teacher and had increased by 1977 to employ six teachers, each with case loads of six children. Eighteen of the children had hearing losses in excess of 70 dB. Each was seen by the itinerant teacher for 40–45 minutes four or five times each week. One of the itinerant teachers[235] felt that, to succeed, severely and profoundly deaf children needed to start their ordinary schooling early and have supporting parents.

The San Diego teachers felt that at the primary school level, their work was mainly on communication skills, but as the children entered high schools, their work was more in the subject content area. The itinerant (or, as they were called, 'travelling') teachers made use of an orientation kit developed by Bitter and Johnston to inform teachers and children in ordinary schools about children with hearing losses.[18] This, they said, helped the children to feel comfortable and make the most of their educational and social opportunities.

Within a 35-mile radius of Portland, Oregon, a total of 11 itinerant teachers and one teacher's aide were employed to assist 92 children in 1977–80. Of these 92, 18 were classified as prelingually deaf children, and all attended their local ordinary schools from kindergarten through twelfth grade. The average case load was approximately eight children, but varying amounts of time were spent with different children, depending upon individual need. By law, the maximum time that could be spent with an individual child was five hours per week. Visits were timed as far as possible so as not to cut into the handicapped child's normal class lessons.

A number of New York City children in the mid-1970s could not be seen by the itinerant teachers in their neighbourhood schools and, in consequence, they had to travel to a central school for tutoring. As in Portland, Oregon, this could be time-consuming and, unfortunately, often required a considerable disruption to the timetable. This problem is also discussed in chapter 6.

Supervision of the work of itinerant teachers

In north London, the head of the school for deaf children was responsible for this supervision but, due to other commitments, was unable to visit the teachers very often. He relied on weekly reports from these teachers and the support teachers, meetings at the school for the deaf at the end of each term and occasional visits to schools with visitors. In New York City, the chairman of the itinerant teachers spent a minimal amount of time with the tenured teachers, but more extensive supervision was given to probationers.[22]

In Milan, the situation in 1980 was similar to that in north London. Itinerant teachers in New Zealand were also rarely seen in the ordinary schools by the supervising principals of the deaf schools, who seemed to rely on meetings at regular intervals and reports from the teachers.

In addition to regular meetings, it is recommended that visits by an advisory teacher or senior colleague should be made to each of the children's schools at least once each year in country areas and once each term in cities.

Interpreters

Where 'total communication'[117] is used in integration programmes in the United States, some authorities employ a person exclusively as an interpreter. He or she usually uses whispered speech and signs and fingerspelling during each class lesson. In other programmes, the children are accompanied by the teacher of the deaf during academic lessons. At the secondary school level, optional classes for normally hearing children in manual communication are sometimes offered.[23]

In most programmes of individual integration studied by the writer outside the United States, 'oral' interpreters using jotter notebooks have been used effectively for certain periods each week. Normally hearing children have also become very helpful silent 'lip-talkers' for the hearing-impaired child; they have learned to speak softly and carefully to the child and to repeat or rephrase material which is difficult to lipread. They also sometimes lend the deaf children their notebooks. In the USA these children are sometimes called 'buddies' and occasionally are paid for their labours.

Dr O.R. Cornett's 'cued speech' is used by interpreters in a number of countries.[238]

Ordinary school teachers

Classroom demonstrations for unhandicapped children and class teachers

V.V. Yater[236] has made useful suggestions to itinerant teachers of the deaf, when children in an ordinary class are being introduced to the problem of hearing impairment, proposing that the class teacher should be present throughout such sessions, and that the handicapped child should be involved in both the planning and the execution of the demonstration. This should include some aspect of hearing, the hearing aid, speech reading or some other interest which the deaf child could explain to his or her classmates.

The *cost* of hearing aids is a useful way of helping ordinary children appreciate that they are important, and this can be compared with the cost of bicycles or footballs. The effect of using the hearing aid has often been demonstrated with aided and unaided speech tests of hearing. (Some years ago, one enterprising eight-year-old hearing-aid user in north Wales was reported to have done quite well each lunch-time by charging his playmates 'a penny a listen'!) Tape recordings of filtered speech, showing the effect of high-frequency hearing loss and gradually filtering out sound above, say, 2000, 1000 and 400 Hertz (Hz) can be most interesting and helpful to the children and the class teacher.

In England, teachers in Cornwall have produced a 'resource pack' for loan to class teachers in ordinary schools. This contains: a sample of filtered speech consisting of material that is interesting to children; tape recordings illustrating listening through a hearing aid and the advantage of listening with the radio link aids; overhead projector transparencies of 'The Ear and How It Works'; lists of sources of other material; and, finally, an offer of a talk to the class by a local teacher of deaf children.

To aid the casual acceptance of the hearing-impaired child, the class's attention can be drawn to the fact that handicaps are very common: 'One child in six has a handicap. Three of you have glasses, I have glasses, too, and John has a hearing aid to help him hear better.'

Lipreading games - saying words without using voice for the class to recognise - can also be effective. The teacher can say that some words are easy and some are difficult to lipread - for example, 'beautiful' is easy but 'gorgeous' is hard - and can demonstrate that 'some people don't move their lips enough, and some move them too much and look funny'. By turning their backs to the class and asking 'Can you lipread me now?' teachers can show that 'some people don't look at the person they are talking to.' They should also illustrate the need to face the light when possible to make lip patterns more clear and make other suggestions.

There *can* be a problem of drawing undue attention to a handicapped child. If the subject is treated matter-of-factly and the teacher makes observations such as 'Our handicaps *can* be a nuisance, but are not the most important thing about us. We just get on with living and playing and working together and forget our handicaps as much as we can,' the children seem able to accept the situation fairly readily. Northcott[165] has quoted a hearing-impaired student who said, 'A difference doesn't matter when you're with friends.'

Further suggestions

(1) Accept the hard-of-hearing child positively. Your attitude will very largely determine that of the class.
(2) A home visit early in the year can be invaluable.
(3) Try to find the handicapped child's strengths and play them up - it is a tremendous help psychologically if he can excel in something.
(4) Try to form the habit of making certain that the partially hearing child is paying attention before you give instructions.
(5) A friend (preferably a bright one!) who sits beside the hard-of-hearing child can be a very great help to him by explaining instructions or work which have not been fully understood.

(6) Try to use as many visual aids as possible.
(7) Blackboard summaries of lessons and overhead projector transparencies are invaluable to deaf children.
(8) Try to remember not to speak with your back to the class.
(9) Speak clearly at a moderate speed.
(10) Try to see that there is adequate light on your face.
(11) If possible, repeat questions asked and answers given by other children – otherwise, the hard-of-hearing child only understands half the conversation.
(12) Encourage him to let you know if he doesn't follow something.
(13) Give him as much opportunity to speak as any other child in the class.
(14) Occasionally whisper a sentence. Say, for example, 'Who is sitting near my table?' This puts the partially deaf child on the same footing as the rest of the class and helps them appreciate his difficulties.
(15) The more time that can be spent individually on these children the better it will be for them. This is very important, and can often be the deciding factor in whether a child can remain in an ordinary school or will have to be given full-time special educational treatment.

(a) Some teachers are prepared to give them a little time out of school hours, particularly for extra reading and language work. *See* Ewing, A.W.G. and Ewing, E.C. (1964) *Teaching Deaf Children to Talk*, Manchester University Press, pp. 162–9.

(b) A number of nursery, infant and junior school teachers manage to keep 'home/school notebooks' for partially hearing children. In these, significant events at home and at school are recorded daily and the books become an invaluable means of establishing a liaison between home and school.

(c) In secondary schools some teachers give up ten minutes or more of a spare period to give individual coaching in school subjects and in general language and remedial work.

Further reading for teachers in ordinary schools and parents

DALE, D.M.C. (1967) *Deaf Children at Home and at School.* London: University of London Press Ltd.

DALE, D.M.C. (1975) *Language Development in Deaf and Partially Hearing Children.* Springfield, Ill.: Charles C. Thomas.

DALE, D.M.C. (1978) *Suggestions to Parents of Deaf Children.* London: National Deaf Children's Society.

EWING, LADY IRENE and SIR ALEXANDER (1961) *New Opportunities for Deaf Children*, 2nd ed. London: University of London Press Ltd.

EWING, LADY IRENE and SIR ALEXANDER (1961) *Your Child's Hearing*, 3rd ed. London: National Deaf Children's Society.

GROHT, MILDRED A. (1958) *Natural Language for Deaf Children.* Washington, D.C.: Alexander G. Bell Association for the Deaf.

HART, B.O. (1963) *Teaching Reading to Deaf Children.* Washington, D.C.: Alexander G. Bell Association for the Deaf.

MORKOVIN, B. (1960) *Through the Barriers of Deafness and Isolation*. New York: Macmillan.
VAN UDEN, A.M.J. (1968) *A World of Language for Deaf Children*. Amsterdam and Lisse: Swets and Zeitlinger.
WARNOCK, M. (Chair) (1978) *Children with Special Needs*. London: HMSO.
YATER, V.V. (1977) *Mainstreaming of Children with a Hearing Loss: Practical Guidelines and Implications*. Springfield, Ill.: Charles C. Thomas.

Normally hearing children

The part which classmates can play in aiding successful attendance in local ordinary schools can be immensely important. Ensuring that the deaf child establishes warm and meaningful friendships at school should be a major aim of parents and teachers in all such integration programmes. These relationships cannot, of course, be dictated by teachers or parents, but both *can* do a number of things to promote them:

- *Dress*. Extra care should be taken to ensure that the handicapped child is appropriately dressed. Hair should be properly cut and styles should follow current trends.
- *Toys* and later *sports equipment* should be of good quality and able to be shared with other children.
- *Books* and *educational materials* should also be carefully selected and be readily available.
- *Manners* should be taught early – for example, just remembering to say 'Please' and 'Thank you' can be a great help.
- *Invitations* to birthday parties, to swimming and sporting activities and so on have all helped to develop and maintain friendships.
- *Placement in class* is very important. Children who sit together often become friends. Some teachers have deliberately placed a hearing-impaired child with boys and girls from his own street or who live not too far from his home. In this way, friendships formed in class can be continued not only in the playground and during lunch periods, but also after school and at weekends. (This has already been noted as a serious deficiency in both special class and special school provision when many children are taken quite long distances to school by bus or taxi.)

Parental participation in the above suggestions for promoting friendships for their children must be carefully and deliberately encouraged by teachers. There have been disturbing findings in some studies such as the one by Bloom, Slade and the writer in 1969–70 (Connor[43]), which indicated that the majority of parents of 60 deaf children, despite an average of 15 previous visits from advisory teachers of the deaf, were doing only a fraction of the things they might have done in helping their children audiologically, educationally and socially.

Remedial teachers

In a number of cases, remedial teachers in ordinary secondary schools have accepted hearing-impaired children on to their case loads. Usually working closely with the itinerant teacher of the deaf, these teachers have done some splendid work and many of their teaching techniques are well suited to hearing-impaired children.[4,5]

In a fact-finding study of remedial education in United Kingdom secondary schools in 1969, Pumfrey and Sampson visited 205 schools and interviewed 264 remedial teachers.[181] Although the labelling of children as 'remedial', 'slow learner', 'maladjusted' and so on was not felt to be in the children's best interests, most remedial teachers appeared to accept the need for selection. In one or two exceptional cases, the number of children requiring remedial assistance was as high as 40 or even 50 per cent, according to the special teachers; the usual number, however, seemed nearer 10 per cent.

Modifications to aid integration

(a) *Withdrawing children from ordinary classes.* Remedial classes were frequently felt to create more difficulties than they solved for the children since the children could become stereotyped and lose stimulation from more able children and also lose respect for themselves (*see* chapter 2). Remedial *teaching*, by extracting children from their ordinary classes at certain times each week, was felt to be much more successful. Sometimes children were withdrawn from the main class but not from the class*room*. This enabled some team-teaching by class and remedial teachers and has been recommended by Courtney,[49] (*See also* chapter 4.)
(b) *Group work.* Small groups of children requiring, say, extra reading or mathematics sometimes went to the remedial teacher's room for the whole period during English or mathematics.
(c) *Setting.* In setting,[139] children join other classes for English or mathematics, for example, according to their attainments. In large schools with adequate remedial staffing this solution was considered very practicable.
(d) *Methods.* Within the classroom, some teachers had found that certain methods would counteract the sense of segregation and would help reassure the handicapped child that he belonged. 'Too much individual teaching tends to make children feel that there is something different about them.' This was sensed when asking the New Zealand children whether they would like more individual sessions (*see* chapter 6).

Home assistants*

Purpose To give assistance in the home to parents of a deaf child at the request of a local education authority.
To give ancillary help in a school or partially hearing unit.
To give support to the parent in helping to overcome the effects of the handicap – thus relieving stress in the home.

Aims To provide a home assistant – a cross between a health visitor and teacher/social worker – who will give support to the parent of a deaf child, using their own knowledge and experience to help parents over the adverse effects of the handicap.
To provide a voluntary service which the professional worker may call on in working with the deaf child and his or her family.

Volunteers Mothers of deaf children whose own children are now sufficiently grown up to enable them to give help to others facing the handicap for the first time.

Criteria for selection

The volunteer must be:

(1) Free of personal worries (as far as this is ever possible) regarding her own child's education and welfare.

(2) Not be too emotional over the handicap of deafness in a child.

(3) Able to work with, and be directed by, local education and social service officers.

(4) Willing to be 'hired' and 'fired' by local authority officers.

(5) Able to give help to others without direct personal involvement.

(6) Strong enough to accept decisions made in the interests of the service.

(7) Agreeable to control directed from National Deaf Children's Society (NDCS) Head Office.

Qualifications of volunteers

None. Volunteers are known as 'dogsbodies' which is the role envisaged to be taken in the home or school. They are not seen as amateur teachers or social workers. No task is considered too menial if it is of genuine help to the mother or child – for example, taking a mother and child to do the weekly shopping, helping to prepare a meal, doing some ironing, looking after a deaf child (and a brother or sister) while the mother does some shopping, reading a story to the children, *listening* to the mother

---

* This proposal has been put into operation by the National Deaf Children's Society in co-operation with the writer, and first appeared in the summer 1975 issue of *Talk* magazine (London: NDCS).

when she wants to talk. In so many ways it is possible for the home assistant to lift a few of the 'last straws' from mothers who may well be becoming frustrated and discouraged.

Interviewers

Members of the NDCS Welfare Group together with the Development Officer from the Volunteer Centre.

Course for home assistants

Held at the Institute of Education, University of London, and elsewhere.

Placements available

Maximum 15 per course.

Duration

One day a week for seven weeks.

Purpose

To give some formal training to volunteers who have no professional knowledge of the handicap or of social work. Information on the advances made in education and social welfare since the volunteers' own experiences is given to help bring them up to date with current thinking.

Lecturers

Professional people interested in the Service, each taking the students through their own particular field, keeping in mind the role of the home assistant (*see* Appendix 13, pages 209–10).

Course expenses

Students' travelling expenses; tutors' fees; administration costs.

Payment of volunteers

None. Travelling expenses only are reimbursed, currently being met by the NDCS either regionally or nationally.

Administration

Responsibility for the Service rests entirely with the NDCS Head Office. Contact with local authority; control of home assistant; organisation of courses.

Follow-up

Each home assistant has direct contact with the Head Office Welfare Secretary where advice can be sought. Head Office reserve the right to withdraw a home assistant if found unsuitable. The home assistant has the privilege to withdraw from the Service or from situations where there is recognised inability to cope.

A re-call of students is made four months after the end of each course for discussion with lecturers.

Refresher courses in the form of residential weekends will be available.

Local authority

Each authority where there is a home assistant willing to be of service will be notified of the existence of this facility. Wherever possible,

NDCS make personal contact at the request of the interested authority to discuss the administration of the scheme and its potential. If the scheme is acceptable in principle, the authority then interviews the home assistant for suitability.

Amount of intervention

Virtually all children with defective hearing require *some* regular educational support when they are individually integrated in ordinary schools. This is true of those with even very slight hearing losses.[170] It has also been shown that some students require very much more assistance than others (Table 10). In addition, size of class, abilities of teachers, timetable constrictions and the availability of audio-visual aids and other educational materials can also affect the amount of time needed for individual assistance.

After all the above factors have been taken into consideration, it is usually fairly easy for experienced teachers of deaf children to decide with class teachers just how much help will be required for each child. The amount and type of assistance should, of course, be kept under constant review and, as suggested in the Warnock Report[232], very carefully assessed at the end of each school year.

Finance

One important problem which has been raised regularly by officers of many education authorities in Great Britain is that of finance for staffing this new development. All-too-brief reference is made here to this topic. It will be appreciated that if an authority has a large school for handicapped children as well as several units in ordinary schools, it is often difficult to find additional finance to withdraw certain children and place them in their own local schools while still maintaining the special school and units. On the other hand, if an education authority does not have special schools or units for a certain handicap, children requiring special education must be sent to other authorities at considerable expense.

At the outset, a firm commitment to both parents and teachers should be made by education authorities that individual-integration programmes will not, of course, be introduced simply as a means of saving money. Indeed, it is likely to cost a little more in the initial stages if an education authority has units and schools for hearing impaired children while these are all still functioning.

One factor which is clear from observations in all areas and from Table 10, is that the most able children in both schools and units for the hearing-impaired require a great deal less assistance than those who are more severely handicapped. In consequence, it is reasonable and practical to move these children back into their local ordinary schools first, and then gradually to

Table 10 Suggested time allocation and cost estimate of individual assistance for eight children of various ages, abilities and degrees of deafness in each child's local ordinary school, 1977

CHILD	AGE IN YEARS	HEARING LOSS (*Av. 500, 1000, 2000 Hz*)	ACADEMIC ABILITY (A = very bright E = very dull)	WEEKLY INDIVIDUAL ASSISTANCE: *Teacher of the deaf No. of visits per week Hours*	*Assistant teacher No. of visits per week Hours*	*Welfare Assistant No. of visits per week Hours*	WHERE 'SIMILAR' TREATMENT HAS BEEN OBSERVED	APPROXIMATE ANNUAL COST PER CHILD: *Teacher of the deaf £*	*Assistant teacher £*	*Welfare assistant £*	*Total*
1	5	110	E	3 × 30 min = 1.50	—	5 × 4.75 = 23.75	Isle of Wight, Linkoping, Sweden	210	—	1920	2130
2	8	115	C	5 × 48 min. = 4.00	5 × 75 min. = 6.25	—	North London	560	812	—	1372
3	9	95	D+	5 × 45 min. = 3.75	3 × 90 min. = 4.50	—	North London	525	585	—	1110
4	15	90	C−	5 × 45 min. = 3.75	2 × 90 min. = 3.00	—	North London	525	390	—	915
5	5	80	C−	3 × 45 min. = 2.25	4 × 75 min. = 5.00	—	Norfolk	315	650	—	965
6	7	75	B+	4 × 30 min. = 2.00	1 × 75 min. = 1.25	—	North London	280	163	—	443
7	6	60	D	2 × 30 min. = 1.00	3 × 30 min. = 1.50	—	North London	140	195	—	335
8	12	75	C	2 × 45 min. = 1.50	—	—	Norfolk	210	—	—	210
							Wellington, NZ				
							Palo Alto, Calif.				
							N. Sydney, Aust.				
		mean = 87.5 dB	mean = C−					3265	2795	1920	7980
				29 visits	*18 visits*	*5 visits*	* Linkoping children not severely mentally retarded				
Weekly teaching –				19.75	21.50	23.75					
Weekly travelling time –				5.25	3.50	1.25		235	455	80	770
Total hours –				25.00 hours	25.00 hours	25.00 hours					
Annual salaries –				£3500	£3250	£2000		3500	3250	2000	8750
National Insurance (10.75%)				375	350	215					940
Superannuation (9.4%)				330	305	> 12% = 240					875
											10565
Administration (10%)											1057
											£11622

Annual cost per child of individual integration – £1453
Annual cost per child of unit or day school for deaf children† – £2422
Annual cost per child of residential school for deaf children‡ – £3300–£4000

† Inner London Education Authority, 1977.
‡ By 1982, some residential schools for deaf children in the UK were having to charge more than £9000 per child per annum.

transfer those who require more intensive and expensive special educational treatment.

Special education will always be expensive, of course, but once a considerable number of children have been individually integrated, the overall cost can be considerably less than the present-day segregated or semi-segregated practice (*see* Table 10).

10

Assessments

Capable teachers have always been research-minded. It is a sensible procedure to assess where children have arrived in their studies or their behaviour, apply some educational or social treatment for a time and then reassess to help decide how effective one's management has been. The teacher must, of course, keep assessments in proportion. Criticisms of evaluation programmes have included:

- ⋆ Too much testing, for example, testing to no purpose.
- ⋆ Placing undue emphasis on minor differences – either in results or in comparisons of, say, chronological or mental ages and reading ages.
- ⋆ Becoming so 'attainment test conscious' that the whole curriculum can be dominated by them – with serious consequences for other subjects and often for the enjoyment and lasting influence of the test subjects themselves.
- ⋆ Failing to remember that there are other intangibles and aspects of development which cannot be measured by standardised tests. The poet, James K. Baxter, for example, in discussing how difficult it was to assess children's prose, suggested that 'length of essay' was not a valid criterion. He said that perhaps the best piece of writing he had ever received from a child was when an inner-city eight-year-old chewed her stub of pencil for half an hour and finally wrote: 'My brother can lick anyone in this school.'

While bearing the above points in mind, it is also clear that teachers are helped by the periodic testing of their children in certain subjects as they can then plan the amount and level of future work with far more precision. Later in this chapter are listed a number of tests which teachers of the deaf and research workers in England and elsewhere have found useful.

The Hearing-Impaired Stanford Achievement Tests have been used extensively in the annual surveys conducted throughout the United States since the late 1960s by the Office of Demographic Studies at Gallaudet College, Washington, D.C.[101] In his survey of 12 areas of the United States, each with integration programmes for 30 or more severely deaf children, Brill[23] acknowledged that, when the Hearing-Impaired Stanford Achievement Tests were carried out, a few ordinary school class teachers were reported to have given 'inflated grades' to the hearing-impaired children – especially during the first year or two of having the child in their classes. Most teachers, however, seemed to use exactly the same manner of grading for both ordinary and hearing-impaired children.

Assessment for school placement

In the United States and the United Kingdom, placement in a particular educational programme is frequently recommended by a panel of workers and then agreed or rejected by the child's parents. In one school system in Virginia, for example,[23] the selection of school and the placement within the school were recommended by a committee comprising the hearing specialist, the psychologist, the ordinary school principal, a class teacher and also other special educational personnel. If the recommendation was rejected by the parents, the committee suggested the next most suitable placement and so on until the parents' wishes were met. Each child's progress was reviewed annually and transfers could be made if these were felt to be necessary. As far as possible, however, each child was placed in the programme that best met his or her needs and there was not a great deal of transferring.

Educational and personal data schedules

The following interesting rating scale was used by Reich *et al.* in their Ontario survey of 1974–5,[185] and might well be adapted for use by teachers of deaf children with individually integrated, hearing-impaired children. Although more subjective than standardised tests, it clearly takes much less time to complete than the much fuller investigations outlined later in this chapter.

Teacher rating scales

You are asked to rate the hearing-impaired child's *comprehension and use of speech*, as compared with children *with normal hearing*.

1 *Comprehension of speech*

The approximate frequencies are as follows:

A	B	C	D	E
5%	25%	40%	25%	5%
Almost normal understanding of speech	Considerable understanding of speech	Moderate understanding of speech	Some, though limited, understanding of speech	Little or no understanding of speech

Circle rating: A B C D E

2 *Use of speech*

A	*B*	*C*	*D*	*E*
5%	25%	40%	25%	5%
Almost normal use of speech	Considerable use of speech	Moderate use of speech	Some, though limited, use of speech	Little or no use of speech

Circle rating: A B C D E

3 You are asked to rate the hearing-impaired child's *educational standard*, as compared with *other children in your class.*

A	B	C	D	E
5%	25%	40%	25%	5%
Well above average	Above average	Average	Below average	Much below average

Circle rating: A B C D E

4 *Pupil participation in class/group discussion*

A	B	C	D	E
5%	25%	40%	25%	5%
Frequent participation	Considerable participation	Occasional participation	Little participation	No participation

Circle rating: A B C D E

5 *Educational potential of home*

A	B	C	D	E
5%	25%	40%	25%	5%
Much above average	Above average	Average	Below average	Much below average

Circle rating: A B C D E

6 *Intelligibility of speech* (rating by investigator)

A	B	C	D	E
5%	25%	40%	25%	5%
Normal	Slight defective	Moderately defective	Considerably defective	Very considerably defective

Note: Scales 1, 2 and 3 are taken from Redgate, G.W. (1964) *Diagnostic tests of reading attainment for deaf children*. Manchester: University of Manchester.

Two tests of speech production*

Speech production test 1: consonants and rate of utterance

Three characteristics of speech: consonant articulation, rhythm and rate of utterance have been found to be of critical importance in achieving intelligible speech (Hudgins and Numbers 1942, Spencer 1970 and Subtelny 1979). The first part of this test assesses the child's ability to say 25 consonants in 25 words, and the second part measures the rate at which these same words are said (Fig. 17, Table 11).

Initial consonants are usually easier to produce than medial or final ones. In consequence, 23 of the 25 consonants tested are in initial positions, one is medial ('meaSure') and one final ('riNG') – since these last two sounds do not occur in initial positions in English. The other consonants have not been tested medially or finally since this lengthens the test and makes it less practical for teachers. (All the consonants can, of course, be placed in these other positions for testing and teaching whenever the teacher so desires.)

Another constraint in constructing this test was the need for ease of administration and scoring. (With a little practice, both parts can usually be given and scored in five minutes.)

To be useful and interesting for young children, the material had to be simple and able to be illustrated. Each child can keep a personal test sheet of the words, and most enjoy colouring in the picture after each test sound is able to be pronounced correctly.

Part 1: consonant articulation

The aim is to give each child the best possible opportunity to say each test phoneme as intelligibly as possible in a word. The tester sits two to three feet away, in the quietest possible situation. Light should be on the tester's face; for example, he or she should be facing the window. One should speak within four to six inches of the microphone of body-worn or speech-training hearing aids, taking care that the microphone does not conceal the speaker's lips. The test sheet is placed in front of the child; the tester smiles and says: 'I want you to say these words' (indicating them) 'with good speech.' The tester points to the first picture and says: 'This is a path.' He/she next points to the word: 'This says path.' 'Now' (looking at the child as he or she watches) 'can you say path?' Two more trials are given after the tester repeats the test word. The microphone is passed from the tester to the child on each of the three occasions. If the initial sound is said perfectly by the child on one or more of the three trials, it is scored as correct.

Treat the next words of the test in the same way. Multiply scores that are correct by four to obtain percentages.

When 40 per cent or more is achieved on this test, much of a child's speech will be intelligible. even to those unfamiliar with the speech of deaf children.

---

* From: Dale, D. M. C. (1982) *Journal of the British Association of Teachers of the Deaf*, **6**, 3.

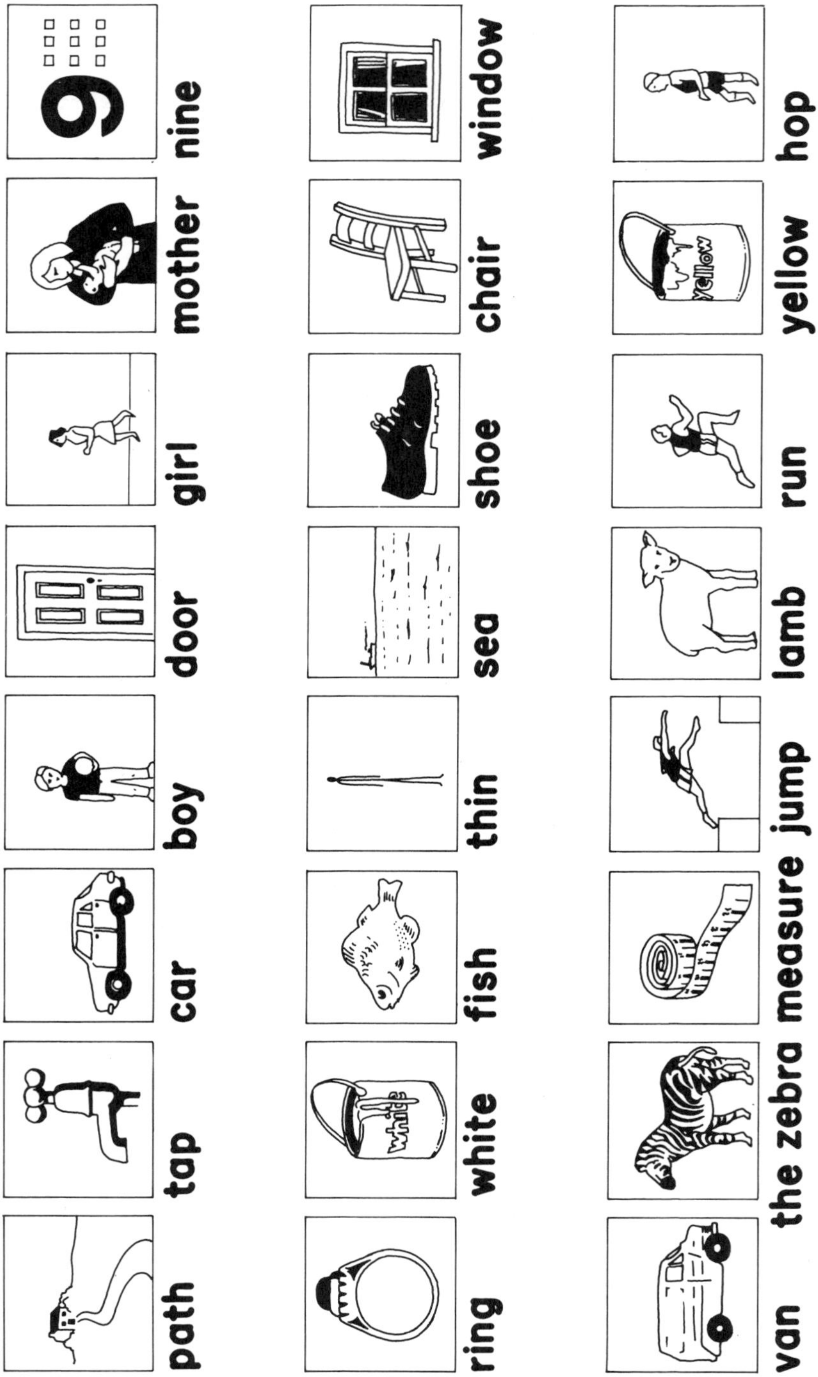

Figure 17 Speech production test of phoneme articulation and rate of utterance.

Table 11 Speech Production Test 1 (score sheet) – Consonant articulation and rate of utterance

Name: ______________________

Date:															
Tester:															
p	path														
t	tap														
k	car														
b	boy														
d	door														
g	girl														
m	mother														
n	nine														
ng	riNG														
wh	white														
f	fish														
th	thin														
s	sea														
sh	shoe														
ch	chair														
w	window														
v	van														
th	the														
z	zebra														
zh	meaSure														
j	jump														
l	lamb														
r	run														
y	yellow														
h	hop														
Total															
×4=%															
Rate Trial 1 Trial 2 Trial 3															
Mean Rate															
Chronological Age															

NOTE. There is a tendency for testers to be too lenient in scoring this part of the test. It is most important to remember that, unless a sound is said perfectly, it should be marked as an error, i.e. 'A good try' is not sufficient. Objectivity is lost if any other criterion is used and results obtained are then of little value.

When used by teachers, results of subsequent tests can be graphed for each child's personal file. As well as being encouraging to both child and teacher, this information can be of real assistance throughout the day. If, for example, a teacher or parent knows that a particular sound can be produced perfectly on one of three trials, he or she knows whether it is reasonable to encourage its use when the child is speaking on some other occasions during the day.

(In all speech work, it is, of course, important to remember Spencer's homily that 'All teaching should be fun.' Coercion or continual nagging is usually counterproductive.)

Part 2: rate of utterance

The object here is to measure the rate at which the child reads each of these three lists of words when speaking at his or her normal rate.

Show the child a digital watch or the second hand on a wristwatch; indicate the first list of eight words, and say: 'Now, I want you to say all these words using good speech and don't gabble.' (Demonstrate by saying the first row of eight words in rapid succession.) 'But don't go too slowly either.' (Demonstrate with exaggeratedly deliberate speech.)

'Ready – go.' (Tester moves hand downwards – neither too slowly nor rapidly, i.e., encouraging a normal rate of utterance from the child.)

Record time

After completing all three lists of words, sum the three times, divide by three and record the *mean* rate of utterance.

Normal rates for reading these three lists with good speech are:

5-year-olds: 8.00 seconds
7-year-olds: 7.00 seconds
9-year-olds: 6.00 seconds
Adults: 4.5–5.00 seconds

If deaf children speak more rapidly or more deliberately than this, intelligibility is lost.

Vowels and diphthongs

Due to difficulties involved in assessing the intelligibility of vowel sounds – accent, voice quality, etc. – these have not been incorporated as part of the above test. Seventeen of the 25 words do, however, contain the commoner English vowels and diphthongs and these can be assessed on other occasions.

Testing and scoring (*see* Table 12) are similar to that indicated above for consonants except that the score for the 17 phonemes correct is multiplied by six to obtain an approximate percentage intelligible for vowels and diphthongs.

Table 12 Vowels and diphthongs (score sheet)

		DATE									
		TESTER									
Long vowels:	ar	(cAR)									
	or	(doOR)									
	ir	(gIRl)									
	ee	(sEA)									
	oo	(shOE)									
Short vowels:	i	(wIndow)									
	a	(vAn)									
	ə	(zebrə)									
	u	(jUmp)									
	e	(yEllow)									
	o	(hOp)									
	oo	(fOOt of the runner)									
Diphthongs:	oy	(bOy)									
	i-e	(nInE)									
	air	(chAIR)									
	ow	(windOW)									
	ear	(EAR—on the lamb!)									

Speech production test 2: consonant blends

This test consists of 40 words containing 40 common initial and final consonant blends (*see* Table 13). It is particularly helpful for partially hearing children and older severely deaf children and adults.

The administration of the test is similar to that for Test 1, but no illustrations are used. The subject is simply shown the word and then, while listening and looking, is asked to repeat it three times after the tester. If the blend is said perfectly on one of the three trials, it is marked as correct on the tester's score sheet.

To score, multiply the final score by 2.5 to obtain the percentage correct. It is extremely rare for a hearing-impaired child to obtain even 75 per cent on this test.

Table 13 Speech Production Test 2 (score sheet) – Consonant blends

DATE										
TESTER										
pram										
brown										
play										
blue										
train										
dream										
twelve										
cry										
grow										
clock										
glue										
frock										
floor										
slow										
stop										
skip										
smile										
snow										
speech										
swim										
three										
ban**ged**										
ap**ple**										
ta**ble**										
lit**tle**										
can**dle**										
buc**kle**										
wrig**gle**										
ri**fle**										
sho**vel**										
stream										
scratch										
spring										
splash										
mar**bles**										
bot**tles**										
rat**tled**										
ri**fles**										
mud**dled**										
sho**vels**										
TOTALS										
% (total × 2.5)										

tree

Figure 18 An example from Hamp's Picture-assisted Reading Test (P.A.R.T.).

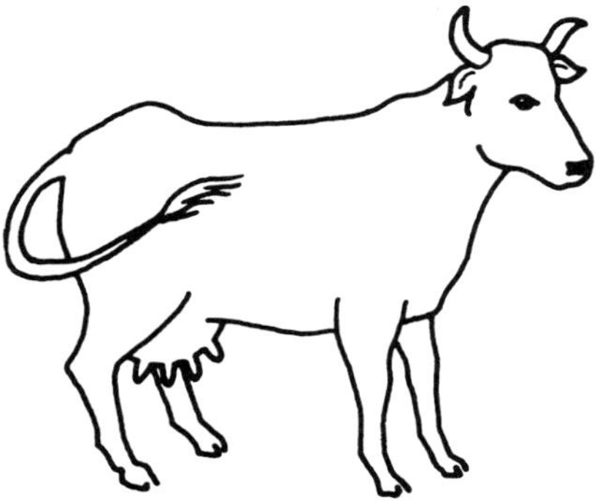

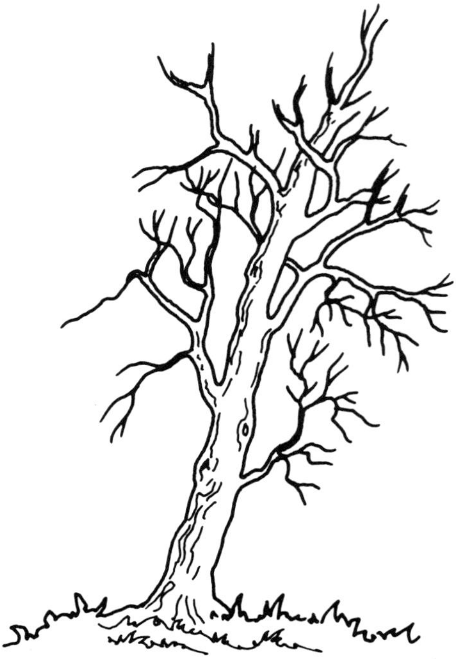

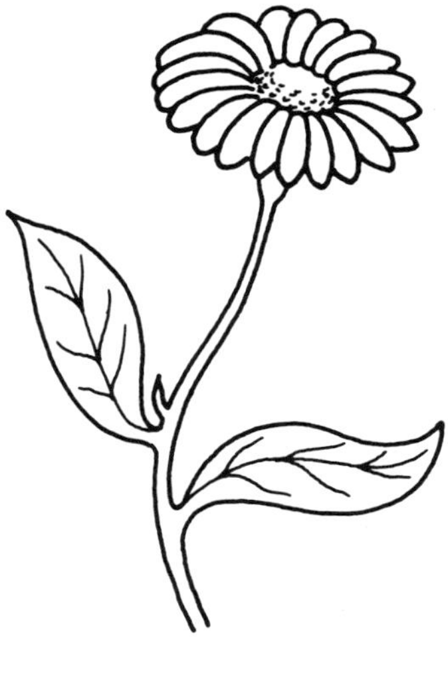

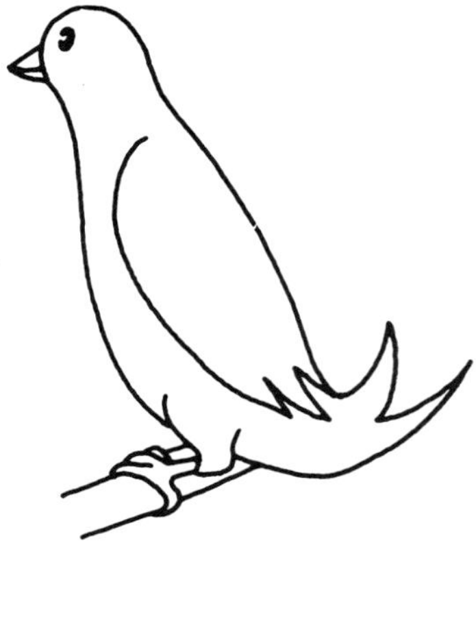

References

1 HUDGINS, C. V. and NUMBERS, F. (1942) Investigation of the intelligibility of the speech of the deaf. *Genetic Psychology Monograph* 25.
2 SPENCER, L. M. (1970) The construction of a test of the intelligibility of speech of hearing-impaired children. Unpublished PhD thesis, University of London Institute of Education.
3 SUBTELNY, J. (1979) Description and evaluation of a training programme to reduce vocal tension in adult deaf speakers. *Volta Review*, **81**, 1–4, 81–90.

Ling's speech acquisition model

A much more comprehensive form of speech evaluation, incorporating speech acquisition, is given by Ling.[141] His 'seven-stage model' is summarised in Fig. 19 (the diamond shapes represent evaluation, and the rectangles represent intervention procedures). The full text is, of course, needed for this model to be used effectively.

Hamp's Picture-assisted Reading Test (P.A.R.T.)

Although other tests are more diagnostic, Hamp's – constructed and standardised by a teacher of the deaf – has proved to be a useful research tool for younger children and very backward readers. It consists of 55 items preceded by the practice items. An item consists of a page on which is printed a word which the child is asked to read aloud. The child then points to one of a series of four pictures on the back of the page which illustrates the meaning of the word (Fig. 18, *see* pp 149–50).

The testing time per child varies from about two minutes in the case of children who are only able to read a few items, to five or six minutes for those who can read most of them. The 55 test items have been graded against groups of normally hearing children, following the principles laid down by Vernon.[229]

The writer has found it useful, before beginning this test with young children or those who are known to be very backward readers, to anticipate the difficulties that will occur. One can turn to items towards the back of the test book and, after indicating one or two difficult words, frown and say, 'These are very difficult, but it doesn't matter – let's read some of these ones at the front.' It has been observed that when the child then begins to get 'out of his depth', he does not feel so upset by failing.

Both deaf and normally hearing children like taking this test as (to begin with at least!) they enjoy the activity of selecting the correct picture from each group of four shown.

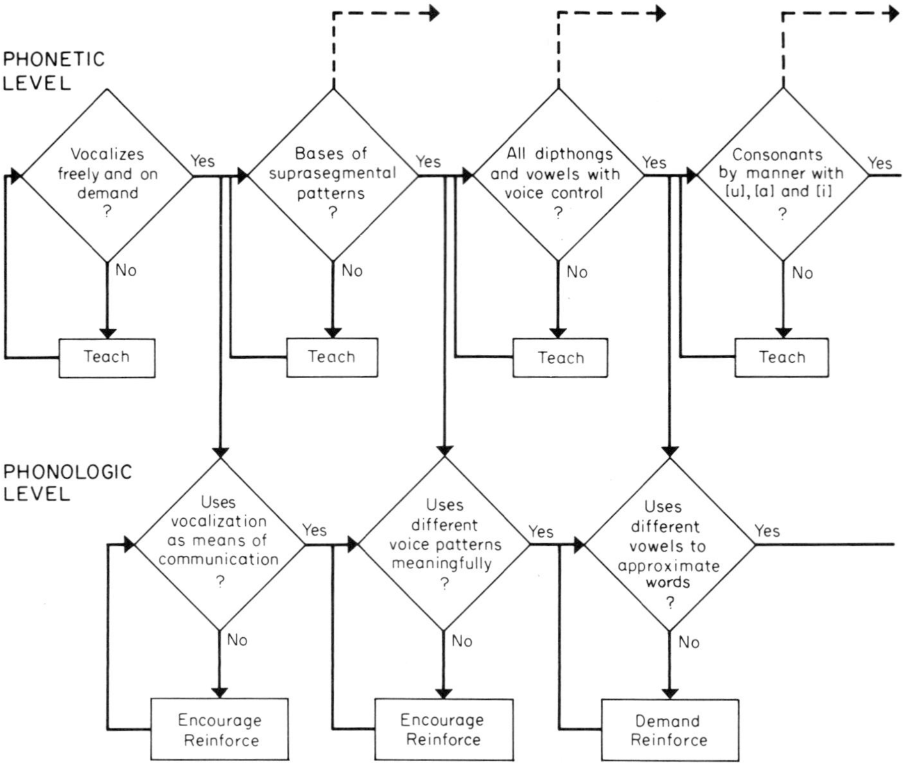

Figure 19 Ling's 'seven-stage model' for speech articulation in hearing-impaired children.[141] (*see* p. 151.)

Daniels and Diack, Reading Test 12

This sentence test involves selecting the correct word, from four or five given words, to make a complete statement. It has proved most useful for testing hearing-impaired children who have a reading age above 7.5 years.

Other tests

The following tests may be used both before and after integration programmes have begun. (The sources for these tests appear on pp. 155–6.)

Audiological

Pre-school

. Ewing Distracting Tests[a]
. Kendall Toy Tests[b]

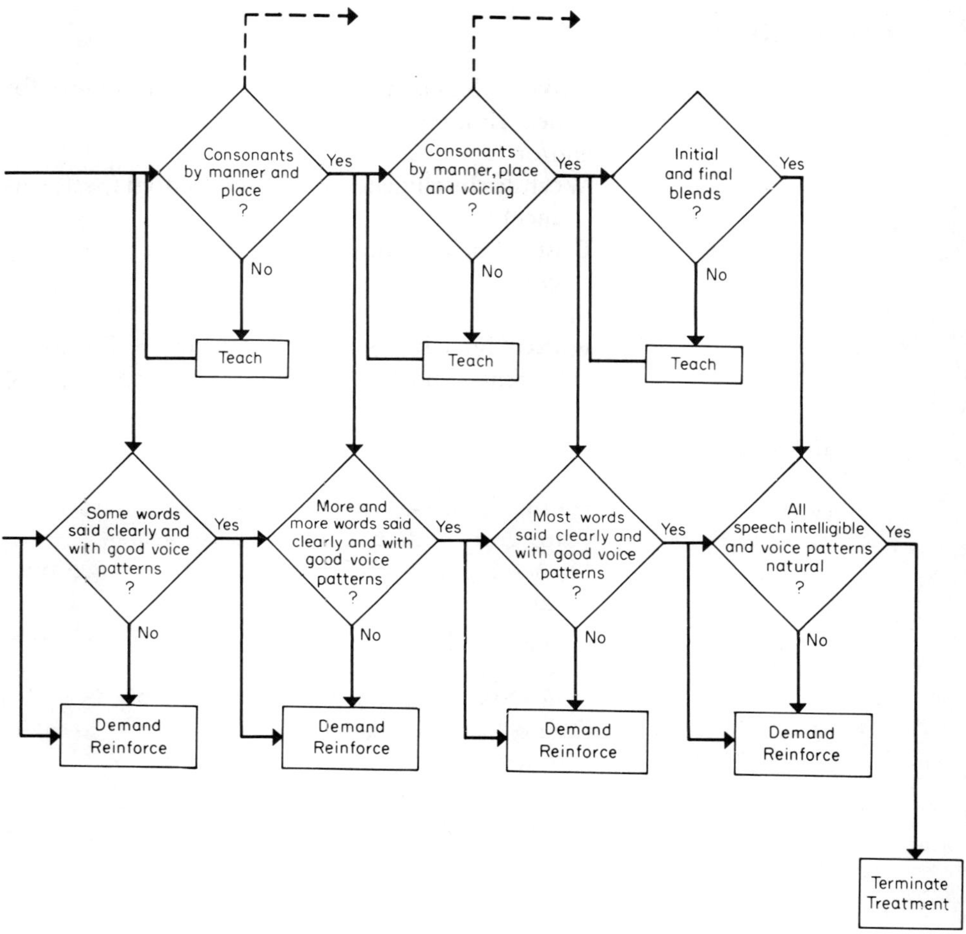

. Peep-show audiometry (from one year)[c]
. Pure-tone air and bone conduction tests[d] (from three to four years where appropriate)
. Impedance measurements[c] (from one year where appropriate)

School-aged children . Impedance measurements[c]
. Pure-tone, air and bone conduction tests[d]

Speech audiometry . Manchester Junior Word Lists[d]
. Consonant Discrimination Tests[f]
. Ten-vowel Discrimination Tests[d]
. Five-vowel Discrimination Tests[d]
. Five-sound Discrimination Test (Ling)[g]
. Paired-vowel Discrimination Tests[d]

'Evoked response audiometry' should be available in the large centres for testing difficult cases (over the age of one year).[h]

Psychological

- . Hiskey-Nebraska Test (test of academic ability for deaf children)
  and/or
- . Wechsler Intelligence Scale for Children (performance)
- . Bristol Social Adjustment Guides[i] (from 5 to 15 years)
  or
- . Rutter Social Adjustment Schedules Forms A (parents) and B (teachers)[j] (from 3 to 15 years)

Educational

Reading	. Hamp Picture-assisted Reading Test[k] (especially for deaf children from five to 10 years)
	. Daniels and Diack, Test 12[l] (for reading ages over seven years)
Speech	. Dale Speech Production – Articulation and Rate of Utterance – Tests (*see* pp. 143–8)
	. Ling's Speech Acquisition Model (*see* pp. 151–3)
Language	. Owrid Language Schedules[m] (from two to eight years)
	. Reynell Developmental Language Scale[n]
Mathematics	. NFER Mathematics Attainment Tests (Forms A and B) 1972[o]

There are, of course, numerous other tests which teachers and psychologists will find especially appropriate for certain children and in certain areas.

Class teachers, itinerant teachers, tutors and others should discuss results of evaluations and implications for future teaching. To help maintain even standards in assessments, and to keep interest alive in the overall findings, and, finally, for their own interest and guidance, it would seem prudent that senior and advisory teachers should also conduct occasional educational and social adjustment tests and ratings.

Suggested time schedules

Audiological testing

Appropriate tests and measurements:

- ★ each year for pre-school children (after satisfactory results have initially been achieved).
- ★ at least every two years for school-aged children.

Hearing-aid performance should be checked when these are serviced by the deaf schools or clinics, and the suitability of aids should be considered at the time of the above tests.

Psychological evaluation

Tests of academic ability should, of course, be administered initially as frequently as the psychologist considers necessary, to establish basic data regarding each child's abilities. Thereafter, each child should be seen routinely every five or six years and more frequently if this is considered necessary.

Social and emotional adjustment schedules should also be administered every five or six years and more frequently if necessary.

Whenever possible, psychologists should take the opportunity to meet parents and teachers and to observe the children in both work and play situations.

Educational testing

★ *Reading tests* for school-aged children should be conducted by senior teachers once or twice each year. These tests are quick to administer and give a most useful indication of overall school progress.

★ *Speech tests:* A–E assessments of overall intelligibility can be made annually for each child since they, too, can be made quickly and act as a minor catalyst.

  Ratings such as the following are quite useful:
  A – Nearly normal
  B – Defective but many intelligible words and phrases
  C – Grossly defective but some intelligible words
  D – Unintelligible
  E – No speech.

  Articulation, rhythm and rate tests should be administered annually to the most seriously handicapped children by senior or advisory teachers and to all children by itinerant teachers, as frequently as is considered helpful, say, weekly for a time, monthly or once each term, depending on the speech programme being undertaken for each child.

★ *Language schedules and assessments* should be completed twice each year for all children up to eight years of age and once each year thereafter.

★ *Mathematics tests* should be carried out twice each year.

References for assessment tests

(a) EWING, A. W. G. and EWING, E. C. (1973) *Deaf Children Under Five*. Manchester: University of Manchester Press, chapter 1.

(b) KENDALL, D. C. (1956) 'The management of deafness in the young child.' Proceedings of the Royal Society of Medicine, 49, 463–7. (See also Dale[50] pp. 38–41 and Appendix 5.)

(c) DIX, M. R. and HALLPIKE, C. S. (1947) 'The peep-show: a new technique for pure tone audiometry in young children.' *British Medical Journal*, **II**, 719.
(d) DALE, D. M. C. (1972) *Applied Audiology for Children*, 2nd ed. Springfield, Illinois: Charles. C. Thomas, chapter 3.
(e) BROOKS, D. N. (1968) 'Clinical use of the acoustic impedance meter.' *Sound*, **2.**
(f) WATSON, T. J. (1972) *Picture-aided Word Discrimination Tests.* Manchester: Department of Audiology, University of Manchester.
(g) LING, D. (1978) 'Auditory coding and recording.' In M. Ross and T. G. Giolas (eds), *Auditory Management of Hearing-Impaired Children.* Baltimore, Md: University Park Press, chapter 6, 195–6.
(h) BEAGLEY, H. (1973) 'Electro-physiological tests of hearing.' *British Journal of Disorders in Communication*, **8,** 115–19.
(i) STOTT, D. H. and SYKES, E. G. (1968) *The Child in School.* London: University of London Press Ltd.
(j) RUTTER, M., TIZARD, J. and WHITMORE, K. (1970) *Education, Health and Behaviour.* London: Longman.
(k) HAMP, N. E. (1975) *Picture-assisted Reading Tests.* Northampton: Arkle Goodman Printers.
(l) DANIELS, J. C. and DIACK, H. (1958) 'Graded test of reading experience.' In *The Standard Reading Tests.* London: Chatto & Windus.
(m) OWRID, H. L. and HAMILTON, P. (1972) 'Comparison of hearing impairment and socio-cultural disadvantages in relation to verbal retardation.' *British Journal of Audiology*, **8,** 27–32.
(n) REYNELL, J. (1969) *Reynell Developmental Language Scale.* Reading: National Foundation for Education Research.
(o) *Basic Mathematics Tests 231, 237, 252, 257* (1972). Reading: National Foundation for Educational Research.

11

Predictive factors which enable successful integration

The following list briefly summarises important factors mentioned in the preceding chapters. It is recognised that it is neither possible (nor desirable) for every factor listed to be checked or provided in the case of every child. A reasonable number of these points should be taken into consideration, however, if one is to expect the programme to be successful. As has already been indicated, when an appropriate hearing aid is fitted and ample daily support from an imaginative teacher, parent or welfare assistant is available, many other factors, although still important, become less critically so. Academic ability, age and personality do, of course, also have high predictive value.

It will be appreciated that all these factors vary from child to child and from one year to the next. For example, one child may have an excellent teacher but a home which cannot offer much assistance, another may have the reverse, and a third child may have a good home and an excellent hearing aid but may be slow in learning. The task of those arranging the support for each child, of course, is to weigh up these various factors - considering the pros and cons in each child's situation - and then provide the degree of support which seems to be appropriate.

1 Selection

It should be remembered that:

(i) *every* child should be considered.

(ii) work for successful placement should begin *six months* before the child begins school.

(iii) where possible, entry should be at the beginning of the school year rather than halfway through.

(iv) the amount of support required depends on a variety of personal, social, educational and audiological factors. For example, young, profoundly deaf children of low intelligence require continuous support from a welfare assistant, and regular visits from an itinerant teacher of deaf children, but older, bright, partially hearing children can often succeed with the minimum of special educational intervention.

Assessments

The following factors should all be taken into consideration when a child is being considered for individualised integration:

Personal
(1) Age
(2) Hearing loss
(3) Academic ability
(4) Personality of child
(5) Amount of support able to be given in the home

School
(1) Head teacher
(2) Class teacher(s)
(3) Remedial teaching available
(4) Class size and composition (e.g., number of children with special needs already enrolled)
(5) Classroom(s): large or small, acoustics, lighting, possibility of tutoring child in classroom.
(6) Teaching aids and materials available to the class
—hardware
—software
(7) Preliminary visit with parents and child - check seating, etc.

Availability of special assistance

Possible assistance from:

* advisory teacher of deaf children
* itinerant teacher of deaf children
* remedial teacher
* welfare assistant
* home assistant/volunteer
* parent
* teacher tutoring before or after school
* classmates

Equipment that will be available to the child:

* radio transmitter
* hearing aid(s) make(s) and model(s)
  earpiece(s) make(s) and no(s)
* speech trainer
* slide viewer
* language master
* textbooks, pictures and other teaching aids

Assistance from parents:
* travel to school (busy roads to cross, etc.)
* checking hearing aids
* home/school notebook
* family diary
* membership of local library
* place for child to do homework
* someone to help supervise homework if parents unavailable
* visiting school for meetings (private and public)

2 One week before entry to school

* Administer appropriate educational and social adjustment tests and schedules (*see* chapter 10).
* Discuss results, first, *briefly* with teacher(s) and then in detail after two weeks, when he/she/they know the child better.

3 Within one month

* Teacher of deaf, class teacher and child to plan a brief lesson on hearing impairment.
* Micro-teaching unit established if possible. Select child's friends and also children living near him or her.
* Home/school notebook begun if possible.
* Child enrolled in local library, accompanied by parent if he/she is unable to do so himself/herself.
* Head teacher/head of department and form/class teacher to attend a one-day session on hearing-impaired children at a teachers' college or centre. Medical, audiological, educational, social and emotional data given – generally and specifically.
* Parents encouraged and helped to visit the school (head teacher to invite them).
* Occasionally, itinerant teacher to take class while class/form teacher tutors the hearing-impaired child.

Reassessments

To be done at the end of Term I and during the second half of Term III, to be followed by conferences of relevant personnel: parents, head teacher, advisory teacher, itinerant teacher, class teacher, psychologist, school medical officer and so on.

12

Recommendations

The recommendations listed below are based on the findings of the work reported in the preceding chapters. It is hoped that these will be helpful to those administering services and to those who care for hearing-impaired children and students, either at home or at school or college.

Main recommendations

1 *All hearing-impaired children and students should be considered for individual integration into their local ordinary schools and colleges.* Evidence has been produced which indicates that a deaf child or college student can integrate much better when he or she is the only deaf person in a normally hearing class (chapters 5, 6 and 8).

2 *Support services for these children and students are essential* in the integrated situation and should be varied according to each child's special needs (chapter 9). Education authorities should be prepared to put adequate finance into this form of education of severely hearing-impaired children and students and at least as much careful planning as has been devoted to segregated provision in the past. Planning each individual child's or student's programme should begin six months in advance of placement (chapters 9, 10 and 11, and Yater[236]).

3 *All local education authorities should consider setting up such carefully planned individual-integration programmes without delay* (chapters 1–11 and Yater[236]). Numbers of children placed individually in their local schools should be restricted in the first year and generous teaching support offered to overcome initial difficulties (chapter 9). Expansion should then be more rapid.

4 *Short initial and follow-up courses of training on individual integration are also essential* (chapters 5, 6 and 9 and appendices 13 and 14). These should be conducted in university departments, teachers' colleges and teachers' centres, and should be for administrators, head and class teachers of both ordinary and special schools and units, advisory teachers of the deaf,

welfare assistants, lecturers in colleges of further education and parents and home assistants.

5 For children who, for one reason or another, are unable to be cared for adequately at home, *residential care in well-supervised 'cottage homes' is recommended*, rather than the traditional hostels attached to schools for deaf children. Wherever possible these children should go home at weekends (chapter 1 and Tizard & Joseph,[219], Tizard & Tizard[224] and Townsend[225]).

6 Irrespective of whether hearing-impaired children and students are taught in special schools or colleges, in units or in individually integrated situations, *every effort should be made to offer regular individual therapy sessions in language, speech, school subject tutoring and in conversations*. Individual treatment has been shown to be far more effective than *group* methods in eliciting oral language from children and students (chapter 1).

7 After very careful preparation of staff and facilities, *many multiply handicapped deaf children can and should be managed in their local ordinary schools* – at least while they are young. Full-time welfare assistants should be engaged to help these children to and from school and throughout the school day (chapter 9).

Further recommendations

8 Small group (micro-teaching unit) sessions are also extremely important for social reasons. Whenever possible, the hearing-impaired child should be joined during these periods by normally hearing girls and boys – if possible, children whose homes are near to him or her, since friendships often develop during such activities which can be maintained after school (chapter 5).

9 Distance education (correspondence school programmes) should be considered to assist individually integrated children and students. These can be particularly helpful for those who are unable to obtain teaching materials at an appropriate level and adequate individual assistance (chapter 9 and Department of Education[70]).

10 Memberships of local hobby, art, sporting and other leisure clubs and societies should be actively sought for each young deaf person who is individually integrated, and pen friends with other deaf boys and girls should also be considered. It is believed that some may also need the company of other deaf youngsters. This is particularly important, if the deaf child has no siblings near his or her own age, and if, after genuine attempts have been made by parents, teachers and social workers, close friendships outside school do not seem easy to maintain between the hearing-impaired child or young adult and his or her normally hearing peers (chapters 1, 5 and 6).

11 Class size and overall ability of the deaf child and other members of the

class are important when assessing the amount of time the class teachers will have available to assist the hearing-impaired child. Where possible, class sizes should not exceed 30 pupils (chapters 1 and 4).

12 Particular note should be made of the type of hearing aids available to each child. Where radio or infra-red transmission can be shown to improve speech discrimination, every effort should be made to provide these – either by the local education authority or by charities (chapters 5 and 6 and Bess,[14] Dale,[50] Huntingdon[119] and Ross and Giolas[191]).

13 Efficient maintenance and servicing of hearing aids is essential (chapters 5 and 6 and Bess,[14] Dale[50] and Ross and Giolas[191]).

14 As a general guide, it is suggested that young, slow-learning, profoundly deaf children from homes which are unable to help them a great deal educationally require a very great deal of special educational treatment. The most important factor seems to be the intelligence of the child – but all factors can be critically important and can affect the amount of special help offered very significantly. Each case should be assessed on its merits, and supervisory staff, class teachers, itinerant teachers of the deaf, parents and the child should keep the levels of intervention regularly under review. It should be remembered that it is possible to *oversupport* a child, but it is much more common to offer too little assistance.

Some staffing requirements and administrative aspects

15 Local education authorities are urged to err on the generous side rather than be parsimonious in staffing these schemes – especially in the early stages and particularly in relation to the allocation of full- and part-time welfare assistants (chapter 8).

16 Where possible, several carefully chosen teachers of the deaf should be appointed and positions of authority allocated so that groups of teachers in a region can act as a team, and supervision and encouragement can be given by experienced colleagues to less experienced teachers, helpers and volunteers (chapters 5, 6, 8 and 9).

17 The head teachers of ordinary schools, although guided by specialist teachers, should take full responsibility for the deaf children who are enrolled in their schools, e.g. for all administrative matters, school progress, social development, and so on (chapters 4 and 6).

18 Where possible, head teachers of schools for deaf and schools for partially hearing children and heads of unit services should maintain professional oversight of children of the type for which they have catered in the past, when these children are individually integrated (chapters 4, 6, 10 and 12).

19 Itinerant teachers of the deaf should sometimes teach the class of ordinary

children while the class teacher spends half an hour or so with the deaf child on a one-to-one basis. This enables the class teacher to become much more aware of the deaf child's problems and strengths and both teacher and child get to know one another much better, which, of course, helps a great deal in future daily contacts between them. The class teacher can then also communicate more effectively with the deaf child's parents. The class of ordinary children then also realise that the teacher of the deaf is a 'real' teacher and not just 'the deaf child's friend' (chapters 4, 5 and 6).

20 Class teachers can sometimes be paid to offer additional coaching to the hearing-impaired child before or after school, two or three days each week. This can also be given by the itinerant teacher of the deaf or some other teacher under the supervision of the teacher of the deaf and the class teacher (chapters 4 and 7).

21 Individual tutoring can also be offered during school hours. At the primary school level, this can be done within the classroom and occasionally in resource rooms, and sometimes singly and sometimes with one, two or three classmates (chapters 3, 4, 5, 6 and 8).

Parents

22 Itinerant teachers of the deaf, class teachers and welfare assistants should all try to establish the closest possible relationships with each child's parents. Home/school notebooks as well as textbooks and assignments are most helpful in maintaining a close and friendly link between home and school and should be conscientiously used.[51,61] Telephone calls have also proved of great benefit to some parents and teachers, and home visits,[51] even though quite brief, can represent one of the most effective means of achieving a strong working relationship between parents and teachers (chapters 9 and 11).

23 Extra time should be taken with *deaf* parents of deaf children when integration programmes are being suggested. It has been found by the writer that accompanying them on visits to ordinary schools to meet the staff and children who will be involved, as well as a careful explanation of the amount of support to be given, will all help to allay the parents' concern (*see* chapter 4).

24 Where welfare assistants cannot be employed, two or three mothers have sometimes arranged to act occasionally as volunteer teachers' assistants. This can be in their own child's class, but can often be in the class of one of the hearing-impaired children of one of the other mothers. (This gives both the mother and the deaf child a rest from one another.)

25 A home assistants scheme (chapter 8) should be examined in each education authority area to ascertain whether or not mothers of older deaf children can be given the opportunity to assist mothers of younger

ones at home and/or at school on a regular, once-or-twice-a-week basis.

26 Teachers of the deaf should help parents arrange occasional small meetings where both parents and children can relax and discuss topics of mutual interest (chapter 9).

Appendices

Appendix I Reading material from an ordinary school class in Milan, used in school by a profoundly deaf boy and taken home

DALL'UOVO ALLA GALLINA

Ero nell'uovo e ogni giorno crescevo un pochino.

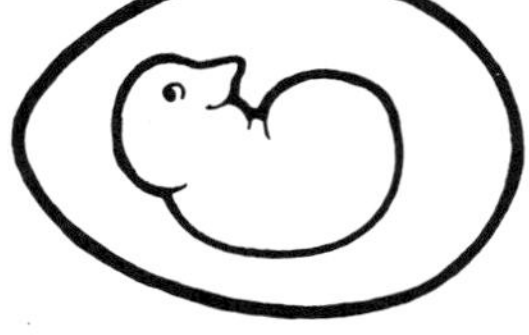

A un certo punto ruppi il guscio e uscii. Ero proprio un grazioso pulcino.

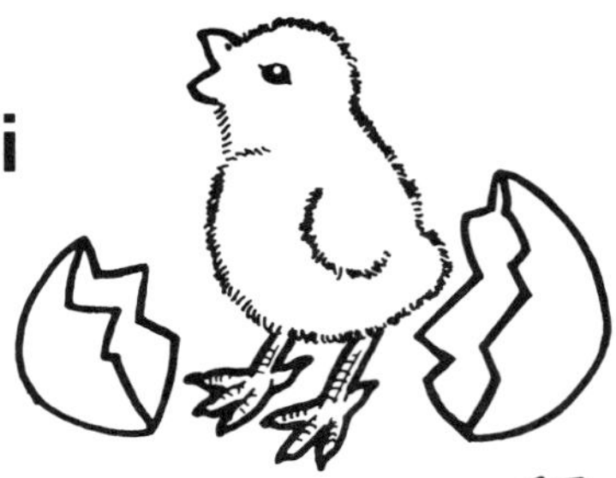

Avevo sempre fame e mangiavo con appetito. Crebbi in fretta e divenni una pollastrella.

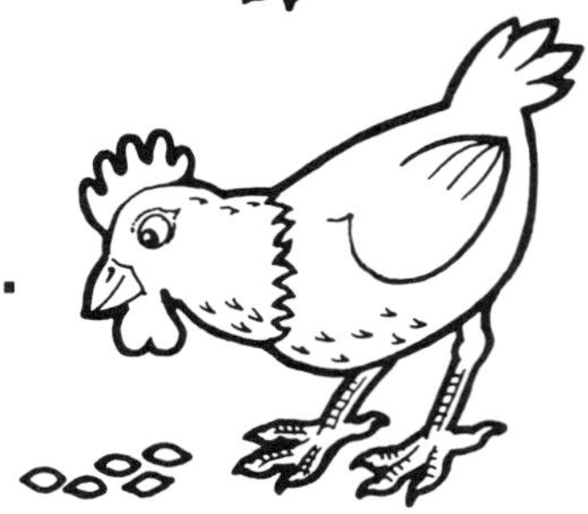

Adesso sono una giovane gallina e so fare l'uovo.

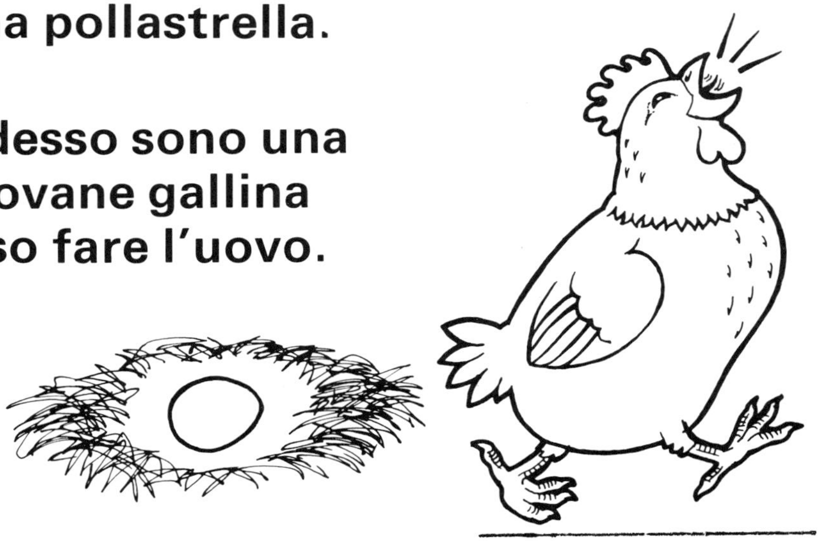

LA GIORNATA DI COCCODÈ

Il  spunta. Al canto del gallo la 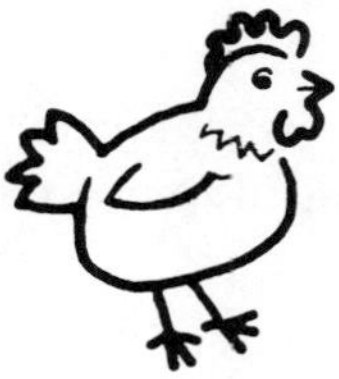 Coccodè si sveglia ed esce subito dal 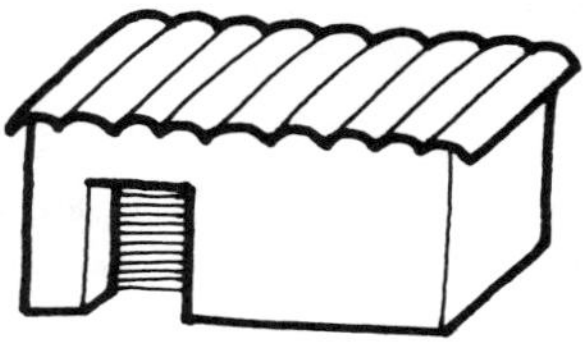

Comincia a mangiare 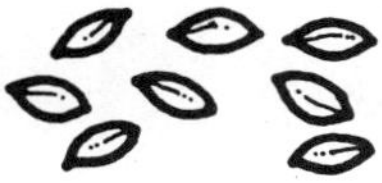 e poi va a bere un po' d'acqua. Infine la 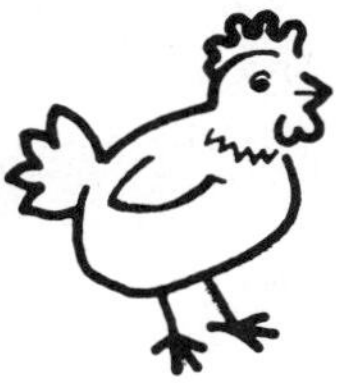 Coccodè si mette a razzolare nel terreno in cerca di 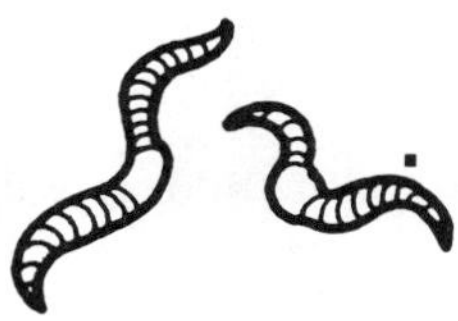. Più tardi depone un 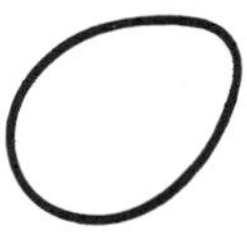 nella cova. Riprende a mangiare e quando il  tramonta entra nel 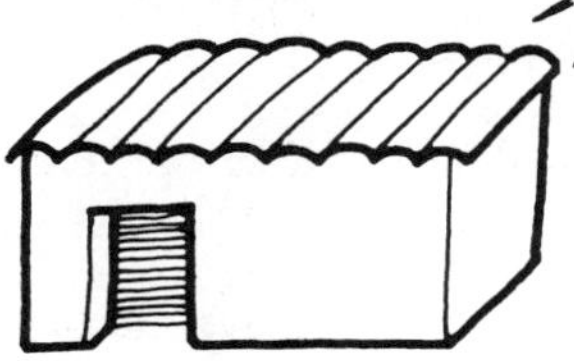 e si mette a dormire.

Appendix 2 Courses for teachers in ordinary schools and parents in Milan, held at the Tarra School for Deaf Children in 1980

Course on 'Problems of verbal communication – integration into the school of a child with language and hearing disorders'

The aim is to make teachers in ordinary schools and public authorities aware of the above and examine the methods of intervention. It is intended to make the course extremely practical.

Course structure
In the first half hour of each session the topic will be set; in the next half hour it will be discussed among the group and in the following hour the lecturers will answer queries. Video-taped material will be used. (The course is taught by teachers of the deaf and lecturers in the education of deaf children.)

Course members
Parents and teachers of ordinary nursery, primary, secondary schools in Milan.

Lectures

1. Concepts of handicap and normality. The child with communicative disorders and disturbances in social environment. His integration into society.
2. Concept of communication. Non-verbal language and communication disturbances.
3. General description of children with communication disturbances. Physical and neuro-handicapped (spasticity and other cerebral lesions); sensory handicapped (hearing-impaired); mentally handicapped (including Down's syndrome); psychically handicapped (neurotic and psychotic disturbances).
4. The deaf child: technical aspects. Deafness, audiograms, prosthesis.
5. The deaf child: logopaedic aspects. Hearing and language, re-education.
6. Dynamic psychology and the effect of the 'disturbed' syndrome in communication.
7. Psycho-affective development and the child with communication disorders.
8. Psychomotor processes: theory and practice I.
9. Psychomotor processes: theory and practice II.

Course on 'Psychology and the interpretation of children's drawings'

The aim is to give people who have followed the previous course the chance of going more thoroughly into topics thought useful for pupils in general and handicapped pupils in particular.

Length of the course
$1\frac{1}{2}$ months - one afternoon per week.

Programme of lectures (two-hour sessions)

1. Psychological dynamics and defence mechanisms. Behaviour as communication. The handicapped situation.
2. Stages of affective development and personal maturity. Psycho-affective alterations.
3. Drawing as expression of oneself. Creativity. Bon Homme Test.
4. Children's drawings: stages of development and environment. Spontaneous drawing and diagnosis of personality. Practice on children's drawings. Family Test I and the School Test.
5. The Tree Test. How it is done. Interpretation. Discussion. Practice.
6. Wartegg Test. How it is done. Interpretation. Discussion.
7. Free-drawing Test. How it is done. Interpretation. Synthesis.

Appendix 3 Reading vocabulary ages and speech articulation scores of experimental and control groups

(a) *Experimental Group 1: Results in unit (1972 & 1973) and when Transferred Individually to Local Schools (1973–77)*

Child	Age in Years: June 1977	Hearing loss (Av. 500, 1000 2000 Hz)	Estimated academic ability	Home rating	Reading Age in Years* In unit		Individually Integrated				Consonant Articulation In unit		Indiv. Integrated		Average rate of Utterance (8 syllables)	
					April 1972	May 1973	May 1974	June 1975	June 1976	June 1977	April 1972	May 1973	June 1976	June 1977	June 1976	June 1977
1	14.9	70	C	D	7.6	7.7	8.4	8.8	9.3	11.0*	15	16	22	22	7.50	5.25
2	13.6	75	C+	B+	8.1	8.9	9.9	10.6	11.0*	11.0*	10	13	20	21	5.25	4.50
3	14.6	95	D	D−	7.3	7.6	8.2	8.3	8.4	8.6	4	2	16	15	6.25	5.50
4	14.8	90	C+	D+	7.6	7.6	8.2	8.6	9.6	10.5	12	18	20	22	3.25	3.50
5	14.8	70	C−	D−	7.7	7.7	8.4	8.9	9.6	10.4	18	20	22	23	4.00	3.75
Mean	14.52	79.00 dB	C	D+	7.66	7.90	8.62	9.04	9.38	10.30	11.8	13.8	20.00	20.60	5.25	4.50
S.D.	0.529	11.576			0.288	0.561	0.722	0.902	.854	.885	4.746	5.741	2.191	2.871	1.53	.791
95% CI					7.4 8.0	7.3 8.5	7.8 9.4	8.0 9.4	8.3 10.3	9.2 11.4						

*Hamp Picture-assisted Reading Test has a maximum score of 11.00 years

(b) Control Group 1: Seven children in hearing-impaired units (1972–7)

Child	Age in years June 1977	Hearing loss	Estimated academic ability	Home rating	Reading Age in years*						Consonant Articulation				Average rate of Utterance	
					April 1972	May 1973	May 1974	June 1975	June 1976	June 1977	April 1972	May 1973	June 1976	June 1977	June 1976	June 1977
1	15.9	85	B	B	7.9	8.2	8.2	8.1	8.7	8.8	14	15	23	18	4.75	5.00
2	14.9	75	C	B	7.2	7.4	7.6	7.9	7.9	8.9	10	12	18	17	3.75	3.75
3	14.6	70	C+	B	7.0	7.4	7.6	7.9	8.7	9.2	14	18	22	18	5.50	4.00
4	14.6	75	B	D+	7.1	7.4	7.5	7.9	8.1	8.6	8	12	19	19	4.00	5.50
5	14.6	75	C−	C	6.9	7.0	7.2	6.9	7.5	7.8	10	8	18	14	5.75	5.00
6	14.5	85	D+	C	7.0	7.2	6.8	7.6	7.5	7.7	6	8	15	12	5.75	5.00
7	14.3	85	C+	D	7.3	7.6	7.5	7.4	7.7	7.9	8	8	14	13	6.25	7.00
Mean	14.71	79.00	C	C+	7.25	7.53	7.56	7.80	8.10	8.51	10.00	12.18	18.50	16.23	5.00	5.05
S.D.	0.491	5.803			0.315	0.318	0.426	0.411	0.515	0.604	2.77	3.63	3.31	2.56	1.005	0.986
95% CI					6.9 7.6	7.2 7.9	7.1 7.9	7.2 8.2	7.6 8.6	7.9 9.1						

(*c*) *Nine children in a school for the deaf (1972–7)*

Child	Age in years June 1977	Hearing loss	Established academic ability	Home rating	Reading Age in Years						Consonant Articulation				Rate of of Utterance	
					May 1972	May 1973	May 1974	June 1975	June 1976	June 1977	Dec. 1972	May 1973	June 1976	June 1977	June 1976	June 1977
1	15.9	110	C	A	6.7	7.6	7.9	7.6	8.1	8.3	3	6	9	10	4.50	4.50
2	15.1	95	B	B	6.7	7.6	8.1	8.1	8.0	8.6	10	4	8	11	9.25	8.50
3	14.8	105	C	A	7.0	7.8	7.9	7.8	8.1	8.6	2	4	13	13	5.50	4.75
4	14.1	100	C	C−	6.3	7.2	7.6	7.5	7.8	7.9	5	4	6	13	6.00	5.50
5	14.0	115	D+	B	6.4	6.8	7.0	7.3	7.8	8.3	2	4	7	14	4.50	4.50
6	13.9	105	C−	C	5.9	6.4	7.0	7.2	7.3	7.6	4	8	13	12	6.50	5.25
7	13.6	105	B−	B	7.3	7.5	7.7	7.7	8.2	8.6	6	6	12	18	7.25	6.00
8	13.5	95	C	C−	6.8	7.6	7.8	7.8	8.6	8.3	4	5	15	13	10.00	6.00
9	13.3	100	C	D	5.9	6.8	7.3	7.4	8.0	7.8	3	2	7	7	4.25	6.00
Mean	14.24	103.33	C	B−	6.56	7.26	7.59	7.6	7.99	8.22	4.33	4.78	10.00	12.33	6.42	5.67
S.D.	0.766	6.25			1.34	1.36	1.29	.60	.934	.969	7.07	4.77	9.27	8.59	5.65	3.16

(*d*) *Experimental Group 2: Five children in five ordinary schools*

Child	C. Age June 1974	H. Loss	Estimated academic ability	Home rating	Read. Age		Cons. Corr.		Rate of Utt.	
					1976	1977	1976	1977	1976	1977
1	12.3	100	C–	D	8.3	8.6	18	19	4.5	5.0
2	11.7	85	C–	D–	7.8	8.3	20	21	4.0	3.0
3	8.7	85	B	D+	7.1	7.6	13	18	6.0	5.5
4	7.7	100	B+	D	6.7	7.3	11	15	9.0	5.75
5	7.5	35	C+	D+	6.5	7.3	6	12	8.25	6.75
Mean	9.58	81.00	C+	D	7.28	7.28	13.6	17.0	6.35	5.20
S.D.	2.03	24.36			.728	.712	5.60	3.54	.838	1.39

(*e*) *Control Group 2: Seven children in a junior school unit*

Child	C. Age June 1974	H. Loss	Estimated academic ability	Home rating	Read. Age 1976	Read. Age 1977	Cons. Corr. 1976	Cons. Corr. 1977	Rate of Utt. 1976	Rate of Utt. 1977
1	12.5	60	B	D	7.0	8.0	15	19	4.0	4.25
2	12.5	75	C–	C	6.9	6.9	16	17	5.75	7.00
3	8.7	75	B	C	7.3	7.9	6	8	7.0	6.00
4	8.5	65	D	D	7.1	7.5	15	19	7.75	5.00
5	8.5	65	B+	B	7.6	8.0	16	15	6.75	4.00
6	8.1	105	C	B	6.3	6.9	9	7	8.60	7.00
7	8.0	60	D–	B	6.2	6.6	13	11	9.00	7.00
Mean	9.56	72.14	C	C+	6.9	7.4	12.7	13.7	6.9	5.8
S.D.	1.89	14.64			0.51	0.51	3.62	4.68	1.59	1.95

Appendix 4 Copies of weekly reports on two individually integrated children

Name: Gloria (100 dB from birth; 10 years old)
Date: 21 November 75
Support teacher: J. Pordes

	MONDAY	TUESDAY	WEDNESDAY	THURSDAY	FRIDAY
Current events	Gloria brought some photographs of her mother and herself on holiday this summer.	All-day class visit. We visited the conservation centre in Epping Forest. Gloria thoroughly enjoyed herself, fully participating in all activities.		A party of 3rd and 4th years are going to see the *Nutcracker Suite* after Christmas (evening performance) – Gloria's parents have agreed to her going.	
Reading	Listening–reading–speaking method used on Diary Worksheets based on Tuesday's visit (1) Trees (2) Mammals (3) Nature of the forest.	She was particularly delighted with the animals – voles and mice had been caught in traps and a ferret was brought round to every group. Bark rubbings and leaf rubbings were made and the circumference and height of a tree measured (the latter using a clinometer). The children	Reading involved in selecting information to write up on the visit.	Two poems – 'Mice', 'The Tree'.	Re-read yesterday's poems and discussed 'A Little Mouse' and 'The Red Squirrel'.

	MONDAY	TUESDAY	WEDNESDAY	THURSDAY	FRIDAY
Period 1	Assembly. Mr Purton gave out swimming certificates. Diary.		Began mounting work, to compile a folder on 'Epping Forest'. Description of how to make a bark rubbing and four escarples taken, and we discussed the *difference between* them.	Assembly.	Continued writing the account of visit – looking particularly at *colour* (of leaves, bark, children's woolly hats and scarves, clear blue sky) and the animals (descriptions of appearance, movement habitat, etc.).
Period 2	Addition of fractions – working out common denominator.	Within her group Gloria worked closely with Paulette. Language involved '*difference between*', e.g. mouse and vole; the four trees we were studying – bark, leaf, shape, etc.; clinometer; mammals and birds which live in the forest.		Began writing an account of the visit. Rather than listing the events of the day we concentrated on the walk through the forest (this was the highlight of the day as the children were allowed to run quite freely), movement – children running, kicking leaves, falling down, squirrels darting between the trees, birds swooping down . . .	

	MONDAY	TUESDAY	WEDNESDAY	THURSDAY	FRIDAY
Period 3	Mrs Heaviside (class teacher) spent most of this time preparing the children for tomorrow's visit – looked at the function of various parts of trees, etc.		Leaf rubbings of the oak, silver birch, beech and hornbeam.		Art club.
Period 4	*See* Reading	Swimming (last session)	Music		Handwriting
Social activities especially integration	No particular incidents have occurred during the first ten weeks to indicate that Gloria is having any problems integrating. She continues to participate in all classroom and playground activities quite happily.			Games	Talked about swimming (Gloria very enthusiastic).

Name: Popi (95 dB; 12 years old)
Date: 15–19 Sept. 1975
Support teacher: I Blagborough

Current events	Hearing aid left at home – 'I forgot'. Brought picture of himself in Greece. Brought £1 for savings bank.	Arrived beautifully dressed in full uniform. Returned report slip.	Popi seems very bright today.	Popi's father is going to see him at swimming club tonight.	Excitedly talked about swimming: 'My father come.'

	MONDAY	TUESDAY	WEDNESDAY	THURSDAY	FRIDAY
Reading	Reading back home news. Reading notes made with Popi in geography.	Words for speech tested and sent home. Corrected orally sentences deliberately written wrongly by me. Notes to copy for geography. Notes to copy for science. Instructions for homework.	Story from *Scope Storybook*. Sentences to fill in words.	Part of story from *Scope Storybook*. Sentences to match pictures.	
Period 1	Oral work on holiday in Greece. I write down some of the information. Popi read it back.	*Withdrawn from class* for sequencing exercises. Given a set of six pictures to put in the correct order from a story. Began writing sentences about each. Construction of sentences appalling! Speech: Mrs Whatley.	*Withdrawn from class*. Quick revision of area and introduction of idea of subtracting two areas. This is in preparation for maths today.	Science: evaporation. Steam and water vapour. How rain is formed.	*Withdrawn from class*. Re-did maths homework together as Popi had obviously not really understood.
Period 2	Physical education with class 2 I.	Maths: Mr Purdy. Harder subtraction. Coped very well. Class well disciplined and industrious. Practice work given.	Speech. Geography: why Africa was difficult to explore, i.e. desert, mountains, forests and rapids. Identifying physical features on the map.		Speech: Mrs Whatley. Rhythm of everyday phrases: 'My father's coming.' 'Could I go swimming.' 'How much please?'

	MONDAY	TUESDAY	WEDNESDAY	THURSDAY	FRIDAY
Period 3	Geography: Introduction of position of S. America, Africa, Antarctica and Australia on world map. Colouring these and labelling them. These will be studied this term.	Games.	Art: Mr Gregson.	Speech	Art and craft.
Period 4	*Withdrawn from class*. Preparation for maths. Adding, subtraction and times (long and short). Classmates' spoken and written names. Looked at book about swimming. Introduced sheet of words to do with swimming.	Games.	Art.	Geography: in class without support. Drew map of Africa and coloured land levels.	Art and craft.
Period 5	Speech: Mrs Whatley. Path-tap test of sounds plus some rhythm training.	Geography: finished map. Copied some sentences and filled in the blank spaces.	Music: listening to record and drawing picture.	*Withdrawn from class*. Corrected English homework and maths. Finished sentences to match pictures about a fire. Used language master matching pictures and recorded sentences. Read first part of story,	*Withdrawn from class*. 2nd half of story 'At the Doctor's'. Vocabulary, e.g. waiting room, surgery, prescription. Revision of southern continents for geography.

	MONDAY	TUESDAY	WEDNESDAY	THURSDAY	FRIDAY
Period 6	*Withdrawn from class*. Short and long multiplication. Word connected with swimming, auditory training and comprehension.	Science: From what parts of its body does a dog lose heat? Vitamins. Evaporation and condensation.	Maths: without support teacher. Subtraction of area.		
Period 7	Maths with Class 2I. Subtraction. Demonstration of method by teacher. Practice by pupils.	Copied notes from science book. Many words need explaining during withdrawal time.	*Withdrawn from class*. Set work. Sentences about swimming and swimming equipment. Putting in words. Reading story in preparation for tomorrow.	Maths: enclosing the greatest area in a fixed perimeter. Grasped idea well.	Maths: finding area and perimeter of rectangles.
Social activities especially integration	Upset at lunchtime by boys in a queue for water. They apparently pushed him and he got wet. When I arrived, they were laughing at his speech.	Enquiries from three of the boys in the class as to how much Popi could hear and understand.			Deputy head stopped Popi in corridor and congratulated him on swimming last night – other boys seemed quite impressed.

Appendix 5 Recommendations for individual treatment of 20 children attending units in Norwich, May 1976

First school unit

Child	Hearing loss	Academic ability	Chron. age (years)	Reading age (Hamp)	Suggested time with: Teacher of deaf	Assistant teacher
1	90	C+	4.0	−5.5	2	4
2	120	C+	5.6	−5.5	5	5
3	88	B+	6.4	6.4	3	5
4	115	D+	6.9	5.5	3	10
5	70(S.S.)	C+	7.0	6.6	2	5
6	105	C+	7.4	6.5	3	5
7	110	C	7.5	6.3	5	5
8	100	B	7.6	7.4	5	5

Middle school unit

9	55	C	7.9	6.4	2	5
10	100	B−	8.5	7.5	5	5
11	75	C	8.5	6.8	2	10
12	110	C	9.3	7.7	5	10
13	60	C	9.8	6.9	3	10
14	55	C	10.9	7.4	3	5

County secondary school (already individually integrated)

15	35	C	12.0	11.0	2	—
16	65	C	12.1	10.5	5	—
17	100+	B+	12.7	11.0+	5	—
18	55	C+	12.7	Absent	5	—
19	75(S.S.)	D−	12.8	7.4	5	5
20	40(S.S.)	C−	13.3	8.6	3	2

S.S. = the hearing loss is 'steeply sloping': that is, it is much worse for high frequency sounds.

Appendix 6 Questionnaires used in the New Zealand survey, 1976

CONFIDENTIAL

INDIVIDUAL CHILDREN
ITINERANT TEACHER QUESTIONNAIRE 1

Child's name: ______________________________
Date of birth: ______________________________
School: (During year 1975–6) ______________________
Intelligence A B C D E (A = highly intelligent – E = extremely dull)
Hearing loss (Better ear threshold average of 500, 1000 and 2000 Hz) __________dB
Any other handicaps: ______________________________
____
____

1 Number of visits made to this child each week: 1 2 3 4 or 5

2 Average time spent in individual work each visit: __________

3 " " " with each child in micro teaching unit situation:

4 (a) " " " observing this child during visit: __________
(b) which sessions have proved most worthwhile: __________
____

5 Total time of 2, 3 and 4: ______________________________

6 I feel this is: (i) too much
(ii) a little too much
(iii) sufficient time
(iv) not quite enough
(v) not nearly enough

7 What percentage of the time spent with this child each week individually was devoted to revision of work given by the class teacher(s)? ______________________________

8 What percentage of the time spent with the child individually each week was devoted to presenting work which you had prepared and brought yourself? ______________________________

9 What two topics during this time seem to have been most successful?

____

____

10 The relationship with the child's teacher(s) was

very close
not very close
other

11 This child has received:	a great deal considerable little	educational support from home.
12 This child has received	a great deal considerable little	encouragement and social training from home.

13 How often did you visit this child's home during last year? ___

14 I feel that my school visits have been of

	crucial considerable little	assistance to this child.
15 I feel that home has been of	crucial considerable little	assistance to this child

16 Is there anything else that you feel might be done to obtain maximum co-operation from parents in the educational aspects of this child's upbringing?

____

____

____

17 Other points or observations regarding this child

____

____

____

CONFIDENTIAL

GENERAL
ITINERANT TEACHER QUESTIONNAIRE 2

1 Did you have any specific training for this work? (Apart from your specialist teacher of the deaf training course) YES/NO

2 If YES, give brief details: ____________________

____

3 Do you feel a full year's training course is necessary for this work? YES/NO

4 (i) If YES, why? ____________________

____

(ii) If NO, what type of special training do you feel would be most helpful to itinerant teachers of hearing-impaired children? (State brief content and possible length of course.) ______

____

____

5 Are there any textbooks or other material that you have found particularly helpful in your remedial work with hearing-impaired children? ____________________

____

6 Are there administrative points which you feel should be emphasised when organising such an itinerant service? __________

____

____

7 Overall I have found this work:

Very satisfying personally
Satisfying
Not very satisfying

Comment: ____________________

____

8 Other suggestions, observations or points: __________

____

____

CONFIDENTIAL

ADVISERS INDIVIDUAL INTEGRATION SURVEY

Ordinary teacher training at ______________________College.

1 Teacher of deaf children qualification from
______________________College/University.

2 Advisory training ______________________College/University

3 Other qualifications: ______________________
____

4 Details of any short courses attended: ______________________
____
____

5 Teaching experience:

	Years
Ordinary primary school	________
" secondary school	________
School for deaf children	________
Unit	________
Other ________	________
Adviser	________

6 What earlier teaching experience would you now consider *ideal* for an adviser?
____
____
____

7 What type of special training would you consider ideal for an *adviser*?
e.g. teacher of deaf training; plus a course of one academic year/six months/three months/six weeks

8 Do you feel in-service training courses should be regularly conducted in your area YES/NO
and nationally? YES/NO

	Area courses	National courses
9 If YES, how frequently?	________	________
what duration?	________	________

10 How do you find your present career?

boring
unsatisfactory
on the whole satisfactory
rewarding
extremely rewarding
other

Further comments: ______________________________

____

____

11 Present case load:

pre-school
infant
primary
secondary
tertiary

12 Do you think more advisers are needed in your area? ________

13 How many children are seen by the itinerant teacher? ________

14 How many of these children would you wish to be seen more often? ______________________________

15 Are there any who could possibly do with fewer visits? ______

____

16 How many other children do you feel should have some help from itinerant teachers if they were available? ________

17 Any further comments on Questions 14–16? ________

____

____

____

____

18 On average, how many hours do you work each week? ______

19 Each week I spend on average the following hours on:

(i) Guidance to parents of pre-school children ________
(ii) Guidance to parents of school-aged children ________
(iii) Guidance to teachers in ordinary schools ________
(iv) Audiology clinic work ________

(v) Office work ____________
(vi) Travelling ____________
(vii) Itinerant teaching ____________
(viii) Other (please specify) ____________

____

____

____

20 Ideally, how much time each week, fortnight or month, would you feel necessary to give guidance to average parents of a deaf child of average intelligence:

	If kindergarten or nursery school available	If *no* kindergarten or nursery school available
(i) In the first year of life?	________	________
(ii) in the second year of life?	________	________
(iii) In the third year of life?	________	________
(iv) In the fourth year of life?	________	________
(v) In the fifth year of life?	________	________

21 What have you found your major problems to be in giving successful guidance to parents:

____

____

____

____

22 Which textbooks and other material have you found *most* useful for parents?

____

____

____

____

23 Which textbooks and other material have you found *most* useful for teachers?

____

____

____

____

24 Any further comments? ______________________________

____

____

____

CONFIDENTIAL

HEAD TEACHER/FORM TUTOR/CLASS TEACHER ITINERANT TEACHER SURVEY

Name of school: ______________________________

No. on roll: ______________________________

Child's name: ______________________________

Head teacher/Form Tutor/Class teacher:

1 Compared with other children in the school, I feel I know this child:

not at all well
a little
about the same
a little better
much better

2 How long has this child been at school? ______________

3 How often does the itinerant teacher visit? ______________

4 Do you feel this is sufficiently frequent? ______________

5 Compared with a number of other children in your school who do *not* receive special teaching, how do you rate this child's educational handicap?

(i) much worse
(ii) not much worse
(iii) about the same
(iv) not so severe
(v) not nearly so severe

6 If (ii)–(v), how many children in your school do you feel could profit from such remedial treatment? ______________

7 Does the itinerant teacher ever teach other children as well as the hearing-impaired one?

YES/NO

8 If YES, how often? ______________________________

9 How do you feel about the itinerant teacher service generally?
of doubtful value
probably quite useful
very much in favour

10 How often does the advisory teacher call about this child?

____

11 Do you feel this is:
too often
about right
not often enough

12 How do you feel about the advisory service?
A ______________________________
B ______________________________
C ______________________________

13 Would you appreciate it if the itinerant teacher could teach one or two other children with reading or learning difficulties at the same time as she helps the hearing-impaired child:
YES/NO/OTHER

____

14 Could the itinerant teacher possibly work in the classroom with you?
YES/NO/OTHER

____

15 Does the itinerant teacher ever observe in your classroom?
YES/NO

16 If NO, would you mind if she did?
YES/NO/OTHER

____

17 *Any further comments:* ______________________________

____

____

____

____

CONFIDENTIAL

PARENTS ITINERANT TEACHER SURVEY

Name of child: ______________________________
Address: ______________________________

____

Other children: M/F ___ Age: ___
M/F ___ Age: ___
M/F ___ Age: ___
M/F ___ Age: ___

1 How long has ______________ been going to school? ___

2 How long has he/she been having help from an itinerant teacher? ______________________________

3 Did he/she have a great deal of difficulty before the itinerant teacher was appointed?

a great deal of difficulty
considerable difficulty
a little difficulty
no difficulty

4 And now? a great deal of difficulty
considerable difficulty
a little difficulty
no difficulty

5 Do you think more time is needed with the itinerant teacher each week?

YES/NO/Perhaps

6 What does ______________ like most in school work? ___

____

7 What does ____________ like least in school work? ____________
____

8 Overall would you say ____________ is:
unhappy
slightly unhappy at school
fairly happy
very happy

9 What does ____________ most like doing most out of school? ____________
____

10 What does ____________ like doing least out of school? ____________
____

11 Has ____________ made *close* friendships at school?
YES/NO/Not really close

12 Has ____________ made *close* friendships at home?
YES/NO/Not really close

13 He/she reads at home:
(i) not at all
(ii) occasionally
(iii) quite often
(iv) a great deal

14 If (ii)–(iv), what does he/she read mostly? ____________
____

15 Do you help him/her with reading or other homework after school?
(i) every night
(ii) nearly every night
(iii) occasionally
(iv) never

16 Have you ever kept a family diary? YES/NO

17 Does your child belong to a local library? YES/NO

18 Do you check that the hearing aid is working:

each morning
once or twice each week
rarely
never

19 What do you do to check the aid(s)?

feedback
listen with receiver off
listen with receiver on

20 The other children in the family are:

(i) of little assistance to the hearing-impaired child
(ii) of considerable assistance
(iii) of great assistance

21 Why? ______________________________

____

22 Have you suggestions for improving the itinerant teacher service?

OPEN (the parent is asked the question without any prompting)

____
____
____
____
____
____

CODED (the following prompts are used)

More visits to the school?
More books?
More teaching materials?
More home visiting?

23 Any other comments: ______________________________

____
____
____
____

CONFIDENTIAL

CHILDREN ITINERANT TEACHER SURVEY

Name of child: ______________________________
School: ______________________________

1 How long have you been at this school? ______________

2 How often does Mr/Mrs/Miss ______________ visit you? ______________________________

3 Do you understand the class teacher?
   (i) never
   (ii) sometimes
   (iii) often
   (iv) usually

4 If (i)–(iii), why? ______________________________
____

5 Do you like this school? YES/NO/It's all right

6 Why? ______________________________
____

7 How often do you take homework home?
   (i) every night
   (ii) two or three times each week
   (iii) once a week
   (iv) once a fortnight
   (v) not at all

8 If (i)–(iv), does your mother or father help you with it sometimes? YES/NO

9 Which subject do you like best at school? ______________

10 Why? ______________________________
____

11 Do you like ____________________ coming to school to help you?

not at all
a little
quite a lot
very much

12 Why? ____

____

13 Who is Mr/Mrs/Miss ____________________ ? (Advisory teacher) ____

14 What does he/she come to school for? ________________

15 Who helps you most with your school work:

class teacher
itinerant teacher
head teacher
parents

16 Does your mother or father help you at home with reading? YES/NO

17 If YES, how often? ____________________________

18 Are you taken out of class for your lessons from ________________ ?

YES/NO

19 If YES, do you like being taken out? YES/NO/It's all right

20 If YES, why? ____________________________________

21 If NO, or 'It's all right', what could make it better?

OPEN	CODED
	Take other children out as well
	Take me before school
	after school
	at lunch-times
	teach me in the classroom
	not come at all
	other

22 Do you like wearing your hearing aid?

- not at all
- not much
- it's all right
- I like it
- I like it very much

23 Why? ____

____

24 Can you hear better at home or at school?

- at home
- at school
- no difference

25 Have you (a) best friend(s) in the class? YES/NO

26 If YES, give name(s) ____

____

27 Do you remember being at school before the itinerant teacher used to come?

YES/NO

28 If YES, was it better or worse than now? ______________________

____

29 Why? ____

____

30 Can you name any good friends at home? ______________________

____

31 Have you any other suggestions about how the teachers could help you more? ______________________________

____

____

____

____

Appendix 7 Deaf students and their majors in the United States, 1974

1 *Agriculture* (2 students)
- Flower arranging (1)
- Horticulture (1)

2 *Business and office* (445 students)
- Accounting (46)
- Book-keeping and business machines (5)
- Business administration (84)
- Clerical (47)
- Computer science (10)
- Data processing (88)
- General business (41)
- Key punch (25)
- Office practice (69)
- Office technician (6)
- Secretarial science (15)
- Typing (9)

3 *Communication and media* (219 students)
- Applied and commercial art (43)
- Design technology (2)
- Graphic arts (printing) (95)
- Graphic reproduction (7)
- Graphics technology (5)
- Offset printing (20)
- Photo processing (29)
- Photo science and instrumentation (1)
- Photography (3)
- Production art (2)
- Professional art and design (7)
- Professional photography (4)
- Technical illustration (1)

4 *Construction* (137 students)
- Architectural drafting (18)
- Architectural specifications (1)
- Architectural technology (22)
- Bricklaying (1)
- Carpentry (19)
- Civil technology (23)
- Electrical technology (7)
- Floor covering (1)
- Plumbing (11)
- Sheet metal (34)

5 *Consumer home economics* (34 students)
- Home economics (34)

6 *Environment and natural resources* (6 students)
- Environmental design (4)
- Landscape technology (2)

7 *Health* (52 students)
- Dental hygiene (1)
- Dental lab technology (6)
- Health occupations (2)
- Inhalation therapy (5)
- Medical lab assistance (5)
- Medical records (4)
- Medical technician (11)
- Medical technology (5)
- Mental health technology (1)
- Nurse's aide (3)
- Optical technology (2)
- Orthotics and prosthetics (6)
- Radiologic technology (1)

8 *Hospitality and recreation* (47 students)
- Baking (4)
- Cake decorating (1)
- Commercial cooking (1)
- Culinary arts (4)
- Food administration (1)
- Physical education (34)
- Recreational technology (2)

9 *Manufacturing and industrial technology* (198 students)
- Chemical technology (3)
- Drafting technology (45)
- Electrical engineering (4)
- Electro-mechanical technology (38)
- Electronics (30)
- Industrial arts (1)
- Industrial drafting (1)
- Industrial electronics (1)
- Lab technician (1)
- Machine tool operation (28)
- Manufacturing technology (1)
- Mechanical drafting (13)
- Mechanical engineering (3)
- Mechanical technology (18)
- Numerical control (1)
- Petroleum engineering technology (1)
- Production machine (5)
- Tool and die making (4)

10 *Marketing and distribution* (2 students)
- Fashion merchandising (1)
- Retailing (1)

11 *Personal services* (10 students)
- Cosmetology (7)
- Dry cleaning (2)
- Wig styling (1)

12 *Public services* (73 students)
- Child care aide (2)
- Child care and education (17)
- Early childhood education (1)
- Library science (8)
- Library technology (9)
- Police science (1)
- Psychology/social work (3)
- Social work (16)
- Social work aide (2)
- Sociology/social work (11)
- Teacher's assistant (3)

13 *Trades* (105 students)
- Air conditioning (7)
- Apparel arts (4)
- Boiler maintenance (1)
- Cabinet making (15)
- Commercial dress making (3)
- Custom apparel and fashion design (6)
- Manual skills (7)
- Painting and decorating (2)
- Power sewing (3)
- Small appliance repair (1)
- Upholstery (18)
- Vending machine repair (1)
- Watchmaking (4)
- Welding (32)
- Woodworking and furniture design (1)

14 *Transportation* (80 students)
- Aeronautical engineering technology (1)
- Auto body and frame repair (16)
- Auto mechanics (24)
- Automatic transmission repair (15)
- Automotive apprenticeship (1)
- Automotive technology (4)
- Brakes and wheel alignment (7)
- Diesel and heavy-duty mechanics (3)
- Highway technology (1)
- Motorcycle repair (8)

15 *Arts and sciences* (291 students)
- Art (25)
- Biology (29)
- Chemistry (7)
- Drama (2)
- Economics (3)
- English (36)
- English and literature (6)
- Fine arts (4)
- Geography (2)
- Government (5)
- History (26)
- Mathematics (33)
- Philosophy (1)
- Physics (1)
- Psychology (41)
- Religion (16)
- Social philosophy (2)
- Sociology (52)

Appendix 8 Some post-school courses available in the United Kingdom

These courses are available in colleges of further education (FE), Workers' Educational Associations (WEA), Polytechnics (Poly) and the Open University (OU). Any of them might be of interest to a deaf or partially hearing student when suitable supporting services are arranged. As indicated in chapter 8, tertiary education centres have been pleased to accept deaf students provided adequate support can be provided.

Vocational and semi-vocational courses

	FE	WEA	Poly	OU
Accountancy	X			
Cost and management			X	
Anthropology			X	
Architecture			X	X
Art teaching				
Calligraphy	X			
China painting	X			
Collage	X			
Enamelling and jewellery	X			
Floral decoration	X			
History of art	X			
Metal work, pewter	X			
copper smithing	X			
silver smithing	X			
hall marks	X			
Painting in oil	X			
water colour	X			
portraiture	X			
Photography	X			
Pottery	X			
Sculpture	X			
Biochemistry				X
Biology	X	X		X
Building			X	
Business studies			X	
Chemistry			X	X
Computer studies	X		X	X
Contemporary studies	X	X	X	X
Dietetics			X	
Ecology				X
Economics	X	X	X	X
Education			X	X
Education, economy and politics		X		X
Engineering, civil	X		X	X
electrical	X		X	X
electronic	X		X	X
mechanical	X		X	X
production	X		X	X
Genes and genetics				X
Geography	X	X		X
Geology	X			X
Graphic design			X	
Health education	X		X	X

Vocational and semi-vocational courses

	FE	WEA	Poly	OU
Historical data and social sciences		X	X	X
History – the early Roman Empire and the rise of Christianity				X
Home economics			X	
Industrial management		X		
Industrial organisation		X		
Information science			X	
Inland waterways	X			
International politics and foreign policy		X		X
Landscape architecture			X	
Language and learning	X	X		X
Languages				
English	X	X	X	X
French	X		X	
German	X		X	
Italian	X			
Punjabi	X			
Russian	X			
Spanish	X			
Urdu	X			
Welsh		X		
Language and business studies			X	
Law	X	X	X	X
Librarianship			X	
Management, education			X	
personnel	X		X	
Man-made futures: design and technology				X
Mathematics, elementary	X			X
linear				X
pure				X
statistics and computing			X	X
Mechanics and applied calculus				X
Micro-economics				X
People and work		X		
Personality and learning		X		
Physical sciences		X		
Physics	X			
Playgroups	X			
Problems of philosophy		X		
Psychology		X		
Public health inspector			X	
Quantity surveying			X	
Reading development				X
Regional analysis and development				X
Religion	X	X		
Renaissance and Reformation				X
Research methods in the social sciences				X
Residential care of children			X	
Secretarial training			X	
School and society				X
Science and the rise of technology since 1800				X
Social work		X	X	
Sociology	X	X	X	
Speech therapy			X	
Teacher training				
Art			X	
Home economics			X	
Mentally handicapped children			X	

Vocational and semi-vocational courses

	FE	WEA	Poly	OU
Three-dimensional design			X	
Town planning			X	X
Travel on a limited budget	X			
Unemployment		X		
World poverty		X		
Physical activities				
Archery	X			
Badminton	X			
Basketball	X			
Canoeing	X			
Cricket	X			
Dancing				
ballroom	X			
children's	X			
folk	X			
Medan rhythmic	X			
old tyme	X			
Scottish	X			
square	X			
Dog training	X			
Fencing	X			
Golf	X			
Hockey	X			
Judo, various	X			
Keep fit: men/women	X			
Tennis	X			
Weight-lifting	X			
Yoga	X			
Skilled crafts				
Angling	X			
Boat-building	X			
Boat-handling	X			
Bricklaying	X			
Car maintenance: men/women	X			
Film making	X			
Horticulture	X			
Model engineering	X			
Navigation	X			
Typewriting	X			
Wine/beer making	X			
Woodwork	X			
Liberal studies				
Archaeology, industrial	X	X		
Art appreciation	X			X
Art of the theatre	X			
Art in the twentieth century				X
Astrology	X			
Beekeeping	X			
Birdwatching	X			
Brass rubbing	X			
Bridge	X			
Broadcasting script, presentation	X			
Bureaucracy		X		
Chess	X			
Citizen's rights		X		
Conservation		X		
Environment, local studies	X	X		
Environment and agriculture	X			

Vocational and semi-vocational courses

	FE	WEA	Poly	OU
First aid	X			
Folk song, social history	X			
Individual liberties		X		
Metrication	X			
Pollution		X		
Population explosion		X		
Social inequalities		X		
Courses for the home				
Book binding	X			
Cake decoration	X			
Candle making	X			
Cookery (many variations)	X			
Corn dollies	X			
Craftwork	X			
Deep freezing	X			
DIY or home maintenance	X			
Dressmaking (many sorts)	X			
Embroidery	X			
Flower arrangements	X			
Fur fashion	X			
Home crafts	X			
Lacemaking	X			
Lampshade making	X			
Leather and suede	X			
Machine knitting	X			
Smocking	X			
Tailoring (many sorts)	X			
Tapestry	X			
Drama				
Creative writing	X			
Drama group	X			
Lipreading	X			
Play reading	X			
Public speaking	X			
Speech training	X			
Visual arts		X		
Music		X		
Brass band	X			
Choral singing	X			
Development of instruments and their music	X			
Guitar playing	X			
Music	X			
Orchestra	X			
Organ playing	X			
Pianoforte	X			
Recorder playing	X			

Appendix 9 Interview forms and replies

Principals, directors and secretaries of 11 colleges of further education which had not previously admitted hearing-impaired students, October–November 1974

Name of Institution ______________________________

Date ______________ Interview with ______________________

QUESTIONS	REPLIES
1 Do you think it would be in order for, say, a teacher of the deaf or a social worker to bring a projected student and his/her parents to have a brief look at your college prior to enrolling for a course?	YES 11 NO 0 PERHAPS 0
2 If yes, should such a visit be made during working hours or when students are absent?	DURING WORKING HOURS 11
3 Do you think that lecturers would be prepared to: (a) wear transmitter microphones if a hearing-impaired student was in their class? (b) make a little more use of the blackboard or overhead projector? (c) make a little more use of other visual aids (slides, film strips, etc.) (d) give an outline of the course before it begins? (e) give cyclostyled handouts during the course? 4(a) Do you think that an able student might provide a carbon copy of lecture notes for a deaf student?	All 11 colleges replied YES
4(b) If YES, should such help be paid or unpaid?	PAID 11 UNPAID 0
5 Would you agree (when necessary) to a social worker or teacher of the deaf offering tutorials for deaf students?	YES 11 NO 0 OTHER 0
6 In some cases do you think that an interpreter might sit unobtrusively at the side or back of a class while a lecture or session was in progress, to interpret what was going on for the deaf student?	YES 11 NO 0

QUESTIONS	REPLIES		
7 Do you think your lecturers would be prepared to give one hour	YES	NO	PERHAPS
(a) per week	7	3	1
(b) per month	8	2	1
(c) per term	10	0	1
to work with teachers or interpreters on tutorial work if necessary?			
8 Should 7(a), (b) or (c) be paid or unpaid?	PAID		3
	UNPAID		3
	UNDECIDED		5
9 Would you agree to the linguistic aspects of examination papers being explained to deaf students to ensure that they understand the questions?	YES		10
	NO		1

Appendix 10 Link courses, London

A variety of link courses have been organised by the City Literary Institute Centre for the Deaf in London for final-year school leavers. The courses have been arranged with the close co-operation of a number of London colleges of further education, which have made facilities and staff available in order to accommodate special groups of hearing-impaired students. The majority of the link courses take place between Whitsun and the end of the summer term after the main examination period.

Courses are supervised by members of the Centre for the Deaf staff who, in some instances, combine for 'team teaching' with members of the college staff, in order to assist with communication and language difficulties.

The duration of courses varies according to the nature of the course and the provision which the individual colleges are able to make. The aim of a link course is to provide a 'bridge' and 'taster' for possible trades, careers, or further training, and to give opportunities for acquiring additional skills and to assist with maturation.

The following courses have taken place since 1973:

Office skills: one- to three-day intensive course – preparation for work or for further education.

Commerce: one day per week – taster assessment.

Commerce: block course – preparation for work.

Commerce: one day per week for 32 weeks – commercial skills.

Keyboard skills: three- to six-day course – preparation and assessment for punch-card operators.

Printing trades: three weeks, one-half day per week – taster course.

Printing trades: six to eight weeks, one-half day per week – advanced course.

Furniture trades: 16 weeks, one day per week – trade training and assessment.

Soft furnishings: 32-week trade training course.

Floristry: one-day taster course.
Catering: one day per week for a term - training in catering skills.
Engineering: six weeks, one day per week - trade training and assessment.
Child and family care: one day per week for four weeks - general interest.
Pottery: one-half day per week - GCE O level or leisure activity.
Needle trades: one-half day per week for eight weeks - trade training.

Apart from these small group courses, individual links are made in the following courses at colleges of further education:

Car maintenance
Carpentry and joinery
Cookery
Dressmaking
Embroidery
Engineering
Jewellery
Sports activities

Appendix 11 Hearing-impaired students in the Sheffield Further Education Service 1979–80

Of the 31 hearing-impaired students enrolled in the four colleges of further education, nine came for lipreading or speech conservation classes. The other 22, whose hearing losses are listed below, were ex-pupils of schools or classes for hearing-impaired children. Although attending courses individually, 11 of these had to be tutored in small groups by the two teachers of the deaf due to the lack of time available. They received as much individual assistance as possible during these sessions. The other 11 received on average, one-and-a-half hours per week each on individual language support from one of the teachers of the deaf and a further one-and-a-half hours individual assistance from one of the technical lecturers, who was assisted by the senior teacher of the deaf. It was hoped that an additional teacher of the deaf would be appointed to this service as soon as finance permitted.

Better ear thresholds

Student	*500 Hz*	*1000 Hz*	*2000 Hz*
1	75 dB	90	85
2	90	105	NR
3	90	110	120
4	95	105	115
5	80	80	100
6	45	80	90
7	85	90	90
8	90	95	100
9	85	95	95

Student	*500 Hz*	*1000 Hz*	*2000 Hz*
10	110	110	110
11	NR*	NR*	NR*
12	85	95	115
13	90	100	120
14	100	110	NR
15	55	60	90
16	100	100	100
17	105	110	115
18	90	100	110
19	75	90	105
20	75	80	80
21	95	110	115
22	90	100	100

* NR = No response at maximum level of amplification.

Appendix 12 Distance education

The following are extracts from New Zealand Department of Education primary and secondary school correspondence courses that have been arranged for normally hearing children who are unable to attend school - e.g. those living in remote country districts and those who are long-term hospital cases.[70,118,156]

Many of these courses, or parts of them, have proved very useful to hearing-impaired children. In English, for example, while the remainder of the class are studying some abstract topic in literature, the deaf child can work on some basic language assignment more suited to his or her particular needs.

Modern distance education courses are carefully graded and attractively illustrated which make them of real interest to both the student and the supervisor. Supervision can be given by specialist or class teachers, welfare assistants, parents, or a relative or family friend.

Mathematics Set 17
Today use the cardboard clock,
pencil,
page 16 of this set,
numeral cards.

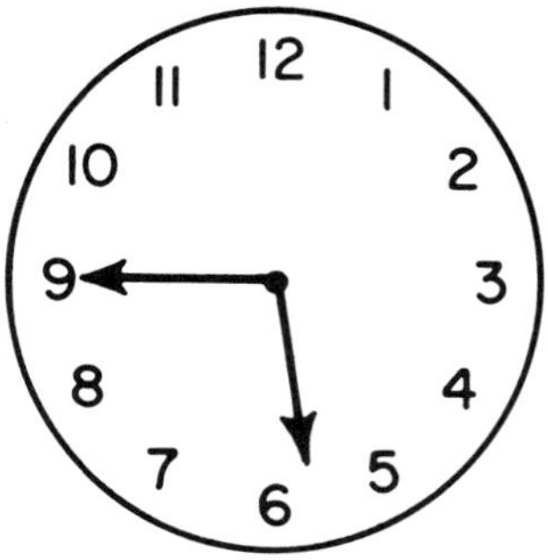

quarter to 6

Everyday Mathematics
Look at the clock.
Can you tell the time?
It is *quarter to 6*
Where does the long hand point? (to 9).
Where does the short hand point? (to just before 6).
Show that time on your clock.
When the *long hand points to 9*
it is always *quarter to the hour*.

You know how
to write *quarter*
as a numeral
like this $\frac{1}{4}$

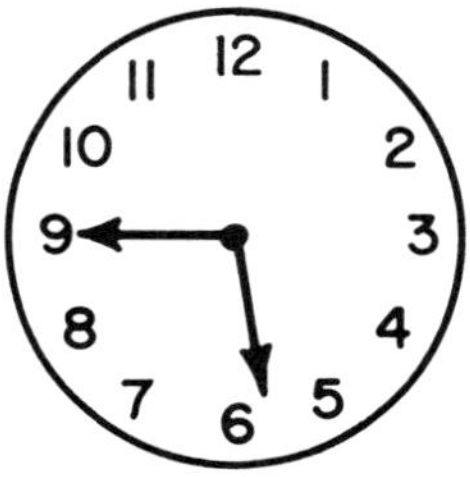

So the time is → $\frac{1}{4}$ to 6

What time is it?
Use your clock to show
and tell Mother each time.
Write a numeral
on each line.

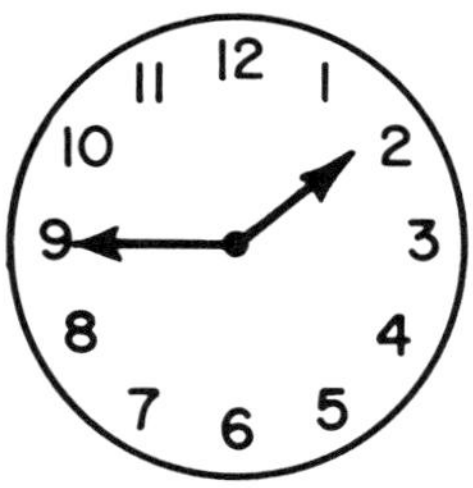

$\frac{1}{4}$ to ___

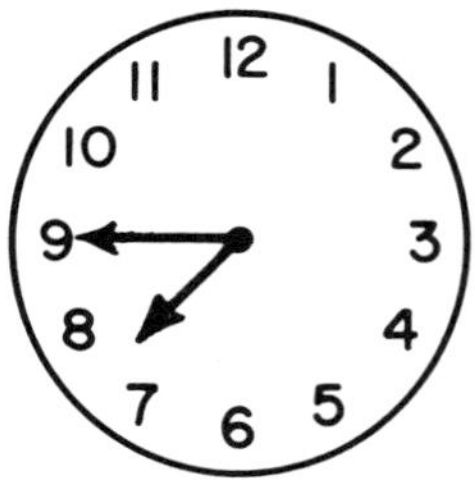

___ to 8

IPS/Sci/9

TEARS AND CRYING

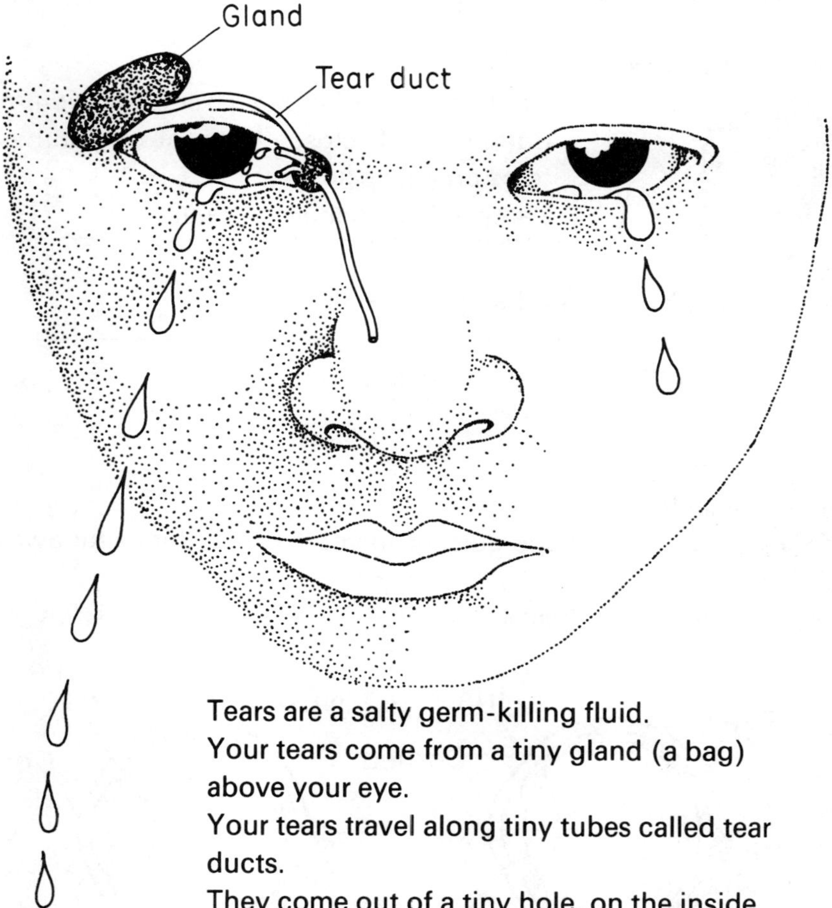

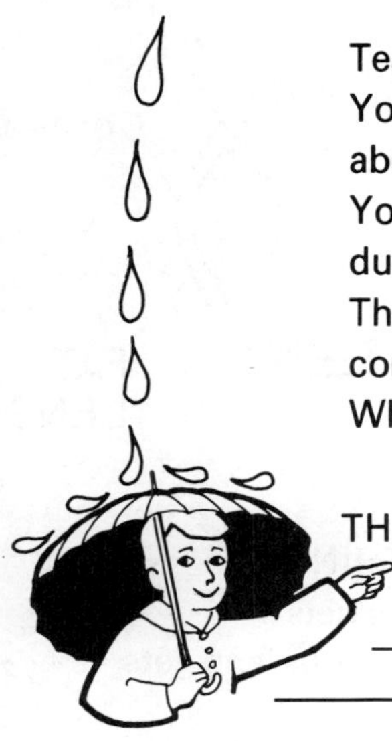

Tears are a salty germ-killing fluid.
Your tears come from a tiny gland (a bag) above your eye.
Your tears travel along tiny tubes called tear ducts.
They come out of a tiny hole, on the inside corner of each eye.
When you blink, tears come out to wash your eye.

THINK If your tear ducts became blocked – what would happen to your eyes?

____

____

IPS/Sci/9

SEEING NEAR AND FAR

Try this if you can:

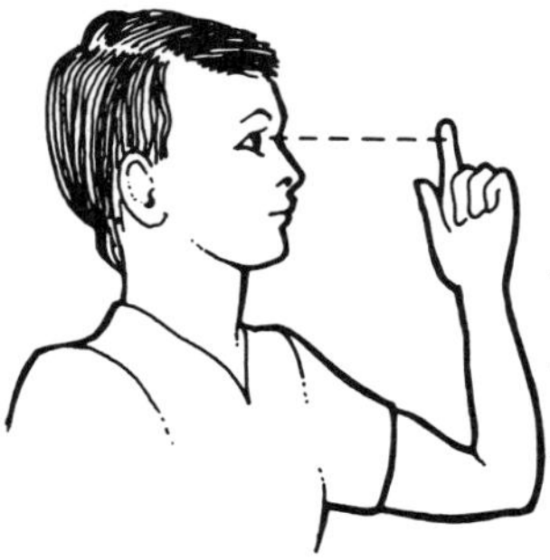

Hold your finger about 15 cm from your eyes. Bring it slowly closer. Keep looking at the patterns on your skin.

Can you feel your eyes strain?

____

What did it feel like?

____

Here's what happens:

Your lens changes shape quickly so you can see things far away, or close to you.

Look at the pictures below:

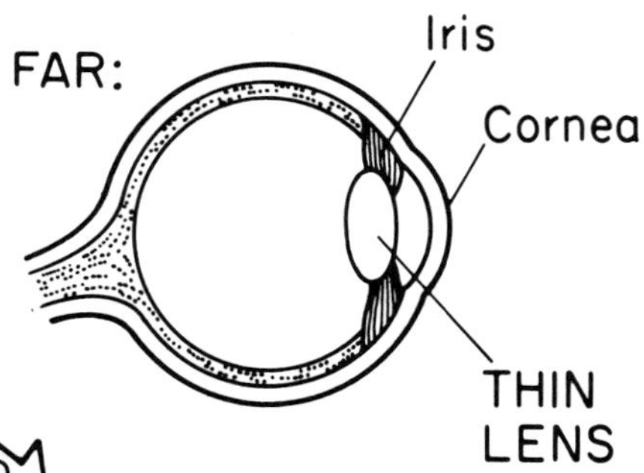

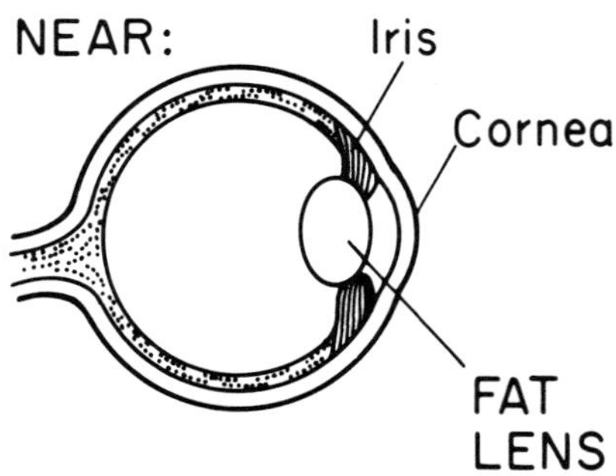

Use these words to fill the gaps: FATTER THINNER

When you look at something far away your lens gets - - - - - -

When you look at something close to your eyes your lens gets - - - - -

PHYSICS/F6/12

PERIODS 9 AND 10

UNIVERSAL GRAVITATION

When it was first proposed that the earth was round like a ball, few would accept the idea. The proponents of the round-earth theory argued that everything is held on the earth by an invisible force called GRAVITY. The earth, they said, is like a great magnet which attracts everything on it, causing stones and other heavy bodies to fall towards the centre of the earth, unless they are held by some means or other. The gravitational force on a body is the WEIGHT of a body.

It was more than a century after Christopher Columbus crossed the Atlantic Ocean and discovered America (1492), before the round-earth theory was generally accepted by thinking people.

Galileo (1564–1642) was a famous Italian mathematician, astronomer and physicist who made important contributions to our knowledge of gravitation and of the planets. He showed that a large cannon ball and a small one when dropped together from a high tower struck the ground together and concluded that, neglecting air resistance, bodies acted on by gravity have the same acceleration. Galileo was the first man to use a telescope to study the skies.

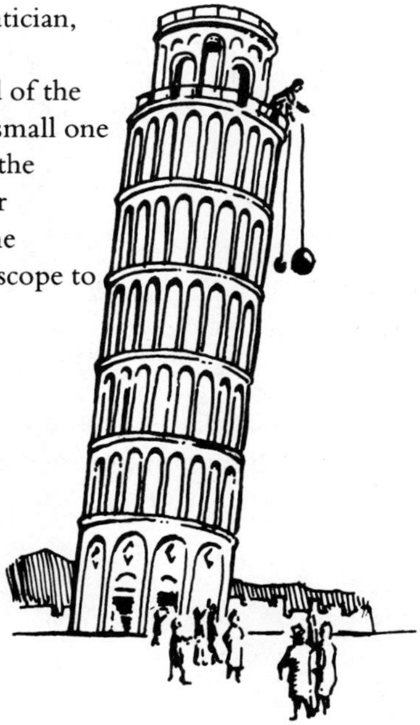

PHYSICS/F6/12

ORBITS ROUND THE EARTH

The MOON is a SATELLITE of the EARTH, while at the same time the EARTH is a SATELLITE OF THE SUN. A satellite is a smaller body which moves in an orbit or path in space round a greater body.
SATELLITES can be launched from the earth's surface to circle the earth, as illustrated below. They are kept in their orbit by the gravitational attraction of the earth.

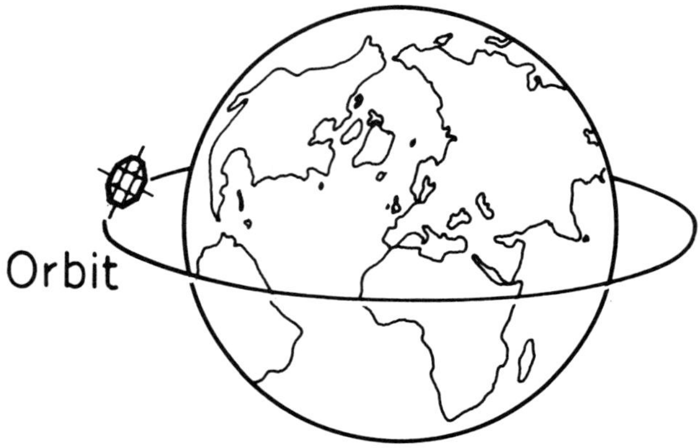

Man-made satellite in orbit

Consider a satellite of mass m which circles the earth of mass M at an average distance R from the centre of the earth at an average speed v.

$$\text{Then } \frac{mv^2}{R} = \frac{GMm}{R^2}$$

$$\text{So, } v = \sqrt{\frac{GM}{R}}$$

If a satellite is in orbit close to the earth's surface it takes about 90 minutes to complete one orbit.

PARKING ORBITS

If the period of the satellite in its orbit is exactly equal to the period of the earth as it turns about its axis, which is 24 hours, THE SATELLITE WILL STAY OVER THE SAME PLACE ON THE EARTH while the earth rotates. This is sometimes called a 'synchronous orbit'. Relay satellites are so placed, so that television programmes, etc., can be transmitted continuously from one part of the world to another.

Appendix 13 Course for home assistants, Bristol, 1976

Wednesday 15 Sept.	10.15 a.m.	Introduction Mrs Freddy Bloom, O.B.E.; Dr D.M.C. Dale, Senior Lecturer in Education of the Deaf, University of London
	10.30 a.m.	Why home assistants? Mrs Freddy Bloom (parent)
	11.15 a.m.	Detection and diagnosis of deafness in children Dr J. Kaye, Senior Clinical Medical Officer, Speech and Hearing Centre, Bristol
	1.15 p.m.	Education of the deaf today – some modern trends and developments Dr D.M.C. Dale
Wednesday 22 Sept.	10.15 a.m.	Pre-school guidance: aims and practice B. McCormick, County Audiologist, Hereford and Worcester Services for the Hearing-impaired
	1.00 p.m.	A handicapped child in the family Dr J. Kahn, psychiatrist
Wednesday 29 Sept.	10.15 a.m.	The young deaf child and his family Dr Susan Gregory, Child Development Research Unit, University of Nottingham
	1.00 p.m.	Videotape (illustrating areas of the morning lecture) Mrs Freddy Bloom; Mrs M. Bennathan, Educational Psychologist, Avon Education Authority; Dr I.M.S. Price, Senior Clinical Medical Officer
Wednesday 6 Oct.	10.15 a.m.	Where will the hearing-impaired child go to school? J. Ashton, Head of External Services for Hearing-impaired Children, Avon
	1.15 p.m.	The role of the home assistant within the educational service Panel representing each area of educational provision; Chairman: D. Williams, Head of Educational Services for the Hearing-impaired, Avon
Wednesday 13 Oct.	10.15 a.m.	Outline of social service provision D.M. Clark, Principal Social Worker in charge of Services for the Handicapped, Avon
	11.00 a.m.	The work of the health visitor An Avon Health Visitor
	11.45 a.m.	Discussion on arrangements for outside visits

	1.15 p.m.	Aspects of social work Miss Celia Davies, Social Worker for Deaf Children and their Families; John Lee, Principal Social Worker, Bristol Institute for the Deaf
Wednesday 20 Oct.	10.15 a.m.	Psychology of deafness: problems of adolescence Mrs M. Bennathan
	1.00 p.m.	Careers for deaf young people Keith Hudson, Teacher in charge of Further Education, Avon
	2.00 p.m.	The young adult The Revd George Firth, The Devon Association for the Deaf
Wednesday 17 Nov.	10.15 a.m.	National Deaf Children's Society responsibility for the Home Assistant Service Mrs B.J. Scott-Ashworth, Director, NDCS
	11.15 a.m.	Open discussion
	1.15 p.m.	Closing panel: discussion Mrs Freddy Bloom; Dr D.M.C. Dale; D. Williams

Appendix 14 Department of Education and Science regional course outline: the integration of handicapped children into ordinary schools, London, 1977–8

Stage 1

Wednesday 21 Sept.	10.00 a.m.	Education of handicapped children in ordinary schools John Fish, HMI, Staff Inspector of Special Education, DES
	11.30 a.m.	Discussion groups
	2.00 p.m.	Historical aspects of the education of handicapped children Dr Marie C. Roe, Staff Inspector for Special Education, Inner London Education Authority (ILEA)
Thursday 22 Sept.	10.00 a.m.	Philosophy of handicap T.W. Moore, Senior Lecturer, University of London Institute of Education
	11.30 a.m.	Discussion groups

	2.00 p.m.	Nurture groups in ordinary schools Mrs Marjorie Boxall, Educational Psychologist, ILEA
Friday 23 Sept.	10.00 a.m.	The education of deaf children in ordinary schools Dr D.M.C. Dale, Senior Lecturer in the Education of Deaf and Partially-hearing Children, University of London Institute of Education
	11.30 a.m.	The integration of visually handicapped children into ordinary schools Mrs J. Kell, Adviser for Special Education, Aylesbury, Bucks.
	2.00 p.m.	The education of children with learning and behavioural problems Tony Staniland, Headmaster, Vernon House, London NW6; Tom Wakefield, Headmaster, Downs View ESN School, Hackney Downs, London E5

Stage 2

Organised locally in the London Borough of Merton to help teachers become familiar with the facilities available.

Wednesday 28 Sept.	4.30–6.30 p.m.	Handicapped children Miss D. Chorley, Adviser, Croydon
Wednesday 5 Oct.	4.30–6.30 p.m.	Assessment and discovery – planning and placing dos and don'ts R.F. Smart, Assistant Director of Education
Wednesday 19 Oct.	4.30–6.30 p.m.	Physically handicapped D. Pettman, headteacher and his staff
Wednesday 2 Nov.	4.30–6.30 p.m.	Integration into ordinary school J.P. Attree, headteacher
Wednesday 9 Nov.	4.30–6.30 p.m.	Support unit Headteacher and staff
Wednesday 23 Nov.	4.30–6.30 p.m.	Visit Miss H. Stephenson, headteacher

Stage 3

Tuesday 29 Nov.	10.00 a.m.	Integration programmes from the school's point of view R. Purton, headmaster, and Mrs Sandra Heaviside, Seven Sisters Junior School
	11.30 a.m.	Mrs H.R. Gould, headteacher, Alexandra Park School, and K. Stroud, headteacher, Alexandra Park Lower School

	2.00 p.m.	R.J. Crosbie, headteacher, Joseph Clarke Special School
Wednesday 30 Nov.	10.00 a.m.	The integration of ESN children into ordinary schools Miss J. Griffith, Paddock School
	11.30 a.m.	Recent research into ways of meeting the needs of physically handicapped children in ordinary schools Dr Elizabeth Anderson, Research Officer, Thomas Coram Research Unit, University of London Institute of Education
	2.00 p.m.	The emotional aspects of handicap in the home and clinic Dr G.S. Udall, Senior Lecturer in Child Health, St Bartholomew's Hospital, London
Thursday 1 Dec.	10.00 a.m.	Parents' attitudes to integration programmes Mrs G. Byrne, Mrs M. Yeoman and Mrs S. Tumin
	11.30 a.m.	Plenary session
	2.00 p.m.	Films: *Growing Together* and *Out of Sight*

Stages 4 and 5 were similarly organised.

Glossary

(definitions of terms as used in this book)

acoustic, relating to the sense of hearing.

aphasia, loss of speech or inability to develop speech which is not due to severe deafness or mental retardation.

audiology, the science of hearing.

audiologist, a person who tests hearing and also frequently advises patients (or their parents) on whether a hearing aid is necessary, which hearing aid to obtain, and how to make the best use of it.

binaural, listening with both ears.

cycle, the three movements of a vibrating object (e.g. a string, reed, or vocal cord) outwards from its rest position, back to a point on the other side, and finally back to its original position.

cycles per second (c.p.s. or Hz), the number of cycles a vibrating object completes in one second.

decibel (dB), one tenth of a Bel. A decibel is the smallest increment of sound that can be detected by the normal ear – i.e. 5 dB can be heard as just louder than 4 dB and 4 than 3 dB, etc. (The word Bel is to commemorate the name of the inventor of the telephone, Alexander Graham Bell.)

diphthongs, sounds which are composed of 2 vowel sounds, e.g. *ie* as in *tie*, *ow* as in *cow*, *ay* as in *day*.

dyslexia, inability to read which is not due to severe deafness or low intelligence.

filtered speech, speech which has had bands of sounds removed. When high pitched sounds are removed, the effect on the speech is often very like the speech of hearing-impaired people who do not produce these sounds because they have not been able to hear them.

finger spelling, using different finger positions to represent the letters of the alphabet. American finger spelling needs only one hand. England and most other countries use two-handed finger spelling. (Many deaf people do not use either finger spelling or sign language, and prefer to communicate orally.)

fundamental pitch, the frequency of the pitch of the voice produced in the glottis.

gain (*of hearing aids*), the amount by which a hearing aid amplifies a sound that is presented to the microphone.

glottis, the 'valve' at the top of the wind pipe, closed off by the vocal cords (or folds).

Hertz (*Hz*), cycles per second. The name commemorates the German physicist who discovered this phenomenon.

high frequency, in voice this can be above 200 Hz for men and above 250 in women. Speech sounds of high frequency are mainly the voiceless consonants such as *s*, *sh*, *th*, *t*, *k*, and *f*, and are mainly over 2 000 Hz in pitch (or, more correctly, in frequency).

peripatetic teachers, teachers who travel about to see deaf preschool children or children with defective hearing in ordinary schools. The word *peripatetic* comes from Aristotle's custom of walking about in the Lyceum while teaching.

References

1 ANTIA, S.D. (1979) 'Education of the hearing-impaired in India: a survey.' *American Annals of the Deaf*, **124**, 758–9.

2 ARNOLD, T. (1888) *The Education of Deaf Mutes: A Manual for Teachers*. London: Wertheimer Lea, Printers.

3 BALLANTYNE, J. (1977) *Deafness*. Edinburgh: Churchill Livingstone.

4 BARATTA-LORTON, M. (1972) *Workjobs*. Menlo Park, Calif.: Addison-Wesley.

5 BARLOW, B. (1975) 'The long-term effects of remedial reading instruction.' *The Reading Teacher*, **18**, 581–6.

6 BATES, A. (1980) 'The integration of hearing-impaired children into ordinary schools' (letter to the Secretary of State for Education). *Teacher of the Deaf*, **4**, 2, 8–9.

7 BEDE, The Venerable. *Historia ecclesiastica* (Book 5, Chapter 2). In T. Arnold (1888), *The Education of Deaf Mutes: A Manual for Teachers*. London: Wertheimer Lea, Printers.

8 BEEBY, C.E. (1966) *The Qualtity of Education in Developing Countries*. Cambridge, Mass.: Harvard University Press.

9 BEGGS HUMPHRIES, M.E. (1959) *The Industrial Revolution 1760–1860*. London: Allen and Unwin.

10 BELLO, J. (1974) 'Curricula and method in education of the deaf in Argentina.' Unpublished report: meeting of twelve international experts in education of the deaf, Unesco, Paris, 30 September–4 October 1974.

11 BELLUGI, U. and BROWN, R. (eds) (1971) *The Acquisition of Language*. Chicago, Ill.: University of Chicago Press.

12 BENNETT, N. (1975) 'The typology of teaching styles in primary schools.' *British Journal of Educational Psychology*, **45**, 20–8.

13 BENNETT, N. and JORDAN, J. (1976) *Teaching Styles and Pupil Progress*. London: Open Books.

14 BESS, F.H. (ed.) (1976) *Childhood Deafness: Causation, Assessment and Management*. New York: Grune and Stratton.

15 BINET, A. and SIMON, T. (1905) 'Upon the necessity of establishing a scientific diagnosis of inferior states of intelligence.' *L'année psychologique*, **11**, 163–91.

16 BIRCH, J.W. (1975) *Hearing-impaired Pupils in the Mainstream*. Reston, Va.: Council for Exceptional Children.

17 BIRCH, J.W. (1974) *Mainstreaming Educable Mentally Retarded Children in Regular*

Classes. Minneapolis, Minn.: Leadership and Training Institute for Special Education, University of Minnesota.

18 BITTER, G. and JOHNSTON, K.A. (1973) *Project NEED for Facilitating the Integration of Hearing-impaired Children into Regular Public School Classes: Final Report*. Salt Lake City: University of Utah.

19 BITTER, G. *et al.* (1973) *Integration of the Hearing-impaired: Educational Issues*. Salt Lake City: University of Utah.

20 BOATNER, M.T. (1959) *Voice of the Deaf: A Biography of Edward Miner Gallaudet*. Washington, D.C.: Public Affairs Press.

21 BOWMAN, E. (1975) 'Mainstreaming hearing-impaired children.' In *Proceedings of the International Congress on Education of the Deaf*. Shinjuku, Tokyo: International Congress on Education of the Deaf.

22 BRILL, R.G. (1978) *Mainstreaming the Prelingually Deaf Child*. Washington, D.C.: Gallaudet College Press.

23 BRILL, R.G. (1975) 'Mainstreaming: form or quality.' *American Association of the Deaf*, **120**, 377–81.

24 BROUGHTON, G., BRUMFIT, C., FLAVELL, R., HILL, P. and PINCAS, A. (1978) *Teaching English as a Foreign Language*, 2nd ed. London: Routledge and Kegan Paul.

25 BROWN, G. (1975) *Microteaching*. London: Methuen.

26 BRUININKS, R.H. and RYNDERS, J.E. (1972) 'Alternatives to special class placement for educationally mentally retarded children.' In E.L. Meyen *et al.* (eds), *Strategies for Teaching Exceptional Children*. Denver, Colo.: Love Publishing Co.

27 BUGLER, J. (1979) 'Revolution in the streets.' *The Observer Magazine*, 98–106.

28 BURMEISTER, E. (1960) *The Professional Houseparent*. New York and London: Columbia University Press.

29 BURNS, A.D. and DAVEY, P.R. (1973) *About the Deaf Child*. Sydney: John Wiley.

30 CALVERT, D.R. (1970) 'The deaf child in the seventies.' *Volta Review*, **72**, 14–20.

31 CALVERT D.R. and SILVERMAN, S.R. (1975) *Speech and Deafness: A Text for Learning and Teaching*. Washington, D.C.: Alexander G. Bell Association for the Deaf.

32 CARLISLE, M. (1980) 'Reply from the Secretary of State to Mr A. Bates.' *Teacher of the Deaf*, **4**, 2.

33 CARVER, V., GILL, J., REID, F. and THACKRAY, D. (1975) *Disability and Assisted Independence*. Milton Keynes, Bucks: Open University Press.

34 CARVER, V. and HALES, G., Department of Special Education, Open University, Milton Keynes. Personal communications with author, 1976 and 1977.

35 CARVER, V., LARGE, P. and LIVINGSTONE, K. (1975) *Providing Supportive Services: The Handicapped Person in the Community*. Milton Keynes, Bucks.: Open University Press.

36 CASTER, J. (1975) 'What is mainstreaming?' *Exceptional Children*, **42**, 174.

37 CASTLE, W.E. (1981) Editorial. *NTID Focus*. Rochester, NY: Rochester Institute of Technology.

38 CHAPMAN, E.K. (1978) *Visually Handicapped Children and Young People*. London: Routledge and Kegan Paul.

39 CHILD, D. and MARKALL, G. (1976) *The Disabled Student*. Eastbourne, East Sussex: Action Research for the Crippled Child and NUS Publications.

40 CLAY, M.M. (1972) *Reading: the patterning of complex behaviour*. Auckland, N.Z.: University of Auckland.

41 CLEGG, A.B. (1970) Secondary school urged to strive for equality: an address on the centennial of the Education Act, 1 May 1870. *The Times* (London), 2 May 1970.

42 CLEGG, A.B. (1968) 'The Newsom Report and its aftermath.' Unpublished. North of England Conference, Education Authority, Liverpool, 3 January 1968.

43 CONNOR, L.E. (ed.) (1971) *Speech for the Deaf Child.* Washington, D.C.: Alexander G. Bell Association for the Deaf.

44 CONNOR, L.E. (1975) 'Mainstreaming the special school.' *Proceedings of the International Congress on Education of the Deaf,* Tokyo, August 1975.

45 CONRAD, R. (1976) 'Matters arising.' In *Methods of Communication Currently Used in the Education of Deaf Children.* London: Royal National Institute for the Deaf 146–55.

46 CONRAD, R. (1979) *The Deaf School Child.* London: Harper and Row.

47 COOK, F. and OCKENDEN, A. (1978) 'Co-operation between schools for the deaf and social workers.' British Association of Teachers of the Deaf (Southern Region) meeting, London, June 1978.

48 COPE, C. and ANDERSON, E.M. (1977) *Special Units in Ordinary Schools: An Exploratory Study of Special Provision for Disabled Children* (Studies in Education 6). Windsor, Berks.: National Foundation for Educational Research.

49 COURTNEY, B. (1978) *The Deployment of Staff in Western Australian Primary Schools. A report.* Perth: Education Department of Western Australia.

50 DALE, D.M.C. (1972) *Applied Audiology for Children,* 2nd ed. Springfield, Ill.: Charles C. Thomas.

51 DALE, D.M.C. (1967) *Deaf Children at Home and at School.* London: University of London Press Ltd.

52 DALE, D.M.C. (1978) 'Educating deaf and partially hearing children individually in ordinary schools.' *The Lancet,* 8095, **II,** 884–7.

53 DALE, D.M.C. (1978) 'L'éducation des enfants sourds et handicapés auditifs integrés dans des écoles ordinaires.' *Le Courrier de Suresnes,* **24,** 2–4.

54 DALE, D.M.C. (1964) 'Integration of deaf children in ordinary schools.' Address to Australian College of Teachers of the Deaf, Hobart, Tasmania.

55 DALE, D.M.C. (in press) 'International perspectives:medical and educational.' In B. Davies (ed.), *Hearing and Hearing Loss* (in press).

56 DALE, D.M.C. (1975) *Language Development in Deaf and Partially Hearing Children.* Springfield, Ill.: Charles C. Thomas.

57 DALE, D.M.C. (1958) 'The possibility of providing extensive auditory experience for severely and profoundly deaf children by the use of hearing aids.' Unpublished PhD thesis, University of Manchester.

58 DALE, D.M.C. (1976) 'A survey of some recent developments in the education of deaf and partially hearing children in ordinary schools and technical institutes in New Zealand.' Unpublished report to the Director General of Education, Wellington, N.Z.

59 DALE, D.M.C. (1973) 'The silence barrier.' *The Guardian* (London), 6 November 1973.

60 DALE, D.M.C. (1971) 'Social aspects of speech.' In L.E. Connor (ed.), *Speech for the Deaf Child.* Washington, D.C.: Alexander G. Bell Association for the Deaf.

61 DALE, D.M.C. (1978) *Suggestions to Parents of Deaf Children.* London: National Deaf Children's Society.

62 DALE, D.M.C. (1982) *A Test of Speech Intelligibility for Hearing-impaired Children. Teacher of the Deaf,* **6,** 3.

63 DALE, D.M.C. (1972) 'Towards individual integration programmes for deaf and

partially hearing children.' In *Proceedings* of the Fourth Danavox Symposium. Elsinore, Denmark. *Scandinavian Audiology*, Supplementum 4.

64 DALE, D.M.C. (1965) 'Units for deaf children.' *The Times Educational Supplement* (London), 3 September 1965.

65 DALE, D.M.C. and HEMMINGS, I. (1971) *Report on Integration Research*. London: Ewing Foundation.

66 DALE, D.M.C. and SLADE, F.W. (1975) 'Post-school education of deaf and partially hearing students.' John Menzies unpublished research report. University of London Institute of Education.

67 DALZELL, J. and OWRID, H.L. (1976) 'Children with conductive deafness: a follow-up study.' *British Journal of Audiology*, **10**, 87–90.

68 DANIELS, J.C. and DIACK, H. (1958) 'Graded test of reading experience.' In *The Standard Reading Tests*. London: Chatto and Windus.

69 DELGARDO, G. (ed.) (1976) *International Directory of Schools and Organisations for the Deaf*. Washington, D.C.: Gallaudet College Press.

70 Department of Education (1980) *The Correspondence School*. Wellington, N.Z.: Government Printers.

71 Department of Education and Science (1967) *Children and Their Primary Schools: A Report of the Central Advisory Council for Education (England)*. London: HMSO.

72 Department of Education and Science (1964) *The Health of the School Child, 1962–1963*. London: HMSO.

73 Department of Education and Science (1974) *Integrating Handicapped Children*. London: HMSO.

74 Department of Education and Science (1979) *Meeting Special Needs*. London: HMSO.

75 Department of Education and Science (1969) *Peripatetic Teachers of the Deaf*. London: HMSO.

76 Department of Education and Science (1978) *Statistics for 1977*. London: HMSO.

77 Department of Education and Science (1976) *Statistics for Education, Vol. 1: Schools*. London: HMSO.

78 Department of Education and Science (1978) *Survey of Behavioural Units*. London: HMSO.

79 Department of Education and Science (1962–3) *A Survey of Children Born in 1947 Who Were Educated in Schools for the Deaf*. London: HMSO.

80 Department of Education and Science (1978) *Report on Education 93: Assessing the Performance of Pupils*. London: HMSO.

81 Department of Education and Science (1967) *Units for Partially Hearing Children: Education Survey I*. London: HMSO.

82 Department of Education and Science & Welsh Office (1977) *A New Partnership for Our Schools: Taylor Report*. London: HMSO.

83 DI FRANCESCA, S. (1971) *Academic Achievement Test Results of a National Testing Program for Hearing-impaired Students*. Washington, D.C.: Gallaudet College Press.

84 D'orientation en faveur des personnes handicapés (1) Loi no. 75–534 du 30 Juin 1975. *Journal officiel, Lois et decrets*, Paris, July 1975.

85 DOUGLAS, J.W.B. *et al.* (1968) *All Our Future*. London: Peter Davies.

86 DUNN, L.M. (1968) 'Special education for the mildly retarded – is much of it justified?' *Exceptional Children*, **35**, 5–22.

87 *Education Act, 1944*. London: HMSO.

88 *Education Act, December 1976* (Chapter 81, Section 10). London: HMSO.

89 Education of All Handicapped Children Act of 1975: Public Law 94–142. *US Code Congressional and Administrative News.* 94th Congress, First Session, **2**.

90 *Education of the Deaf: Report to the Secretary* (1965). Washington, D.C.: Department of Health, Education and Welfare.

91 EWING, A.W.G. and EWING, E.C. (1971) *Hearing-impaired Children Under Five.* Manchester: University of Manchester Press.

92 EWING, I.R. and EWING, A.W.G. (1965) *Speech and the Deaf Child.* Manchester: University of Manchester Press.

93 FARRAR, A. (1901) *Arnold on the Education of the Deaf.* Derby: Francis Carter.

94 FLANDERS, N.A. (1970) *Analyzing Teaching Behavior.* Reading, Mass.: Addison-Wesley.

95 FLINT, B.M. (1967) *The Child and the Institution.* London: University of London Press Ltd.

96 FRANK, A. (1971) *The Diary of Anne Frank.* London: Valentine, Mitchell.

97 *Gallaudet College Alumni Newsletter* (1980) 'Professional day, 19 February 1980.' *Alumni Newsletter,* **14,** 10, 15 March 1980.

98 GARRETSON, M.D. (1976) Committee report defining 'total communication'. *Proceedings* of the 49th Meeting of the Conference of Executives of American Schools for the Deaf, Rochester, NY.

99 GARSIDE, J. (ed.) (1977) *Changing Philosophies and Practices in Education:* a charter for the education of children and adults with handicapping disabilities. Sydney, NSW: Australian Council for Rehabilitation of the Disabled.

100 GENTILE, A. (1973) *Annual Survey of Hearing-impaired Children and Youth.* Washington, D.C.: Office of Demographic Studies, Gallaudet College.

101 GENTILE, A. and DI FRANCESCA, S. (1969) *Academic Achievement Test Performance of Hearing-impaired Students.* (Data from *Annual Survey of Hearing-impaired Children and Youth.*) Washington, D.C.: Gallaudet College Press.

102 GJERDINGEN, D.B. (1977) 'What colleges and universities can deaf children successfully attend?' *Volta Review,* **79,** 112–13.

103 GLYNN, E.L. (1980) *Parents as Remedial Reading Tutors: Report on the Mangere Home and School Project.* Wellington: New Zealand Council for Educational Research.

104 GORMAN, P. (1956) 'I watch his lips.' In Sir Ian Fraser (ed.), *Conquest of Disability.* London: Odhams.

105 GRASER, J.B. (1829) *Der durch gesicht und tonsprache der menschheit weidergegebene taubstumme.* Bayreuth: Frausche, Buchhandlung.

106 GROHT, M.A. (1958) *Natural Language for Deaf Children.* Washington, D.C.: Alexander G. Bell Association for the Deaf.

107 HAMP, N.E. (1975) *Picture-assisted Reading Test.* Northampton: Arkle Goodman Printers.

108 HANEY, R.E. and SORENSON, J.S. (1977) *Individually Guided Science.* Reading, Mass.: Addison-Wesley.

109 HAYCOCK, G.S. (1952) *The Teaching of Speech.* Washington, D.C.: Volta Bureau.

110 HEALEY, W.C. (1977) Foreword. In V.V. Yater, *Mainstreaming of Children with a Hearing Loss: Practical Guidelines and Implications.* Springfield, Ill.: Charles C. Thomas.

111 HEGARTY, S., POCKLINGTON, K. and LUCAS, D. (1981) *Educating Pupils with Special Needs in the Ordinary School.* London: NFER/Nelson.

112 HEGARTY, S. *et al.* (1982) *Integration in Action: Case Studies in the Integration of Children with Special Needs.* London: NFER/Nelson.

113 HEIN, R.D. and BISHOP, M.E. (1978) *An Annotated Bibliography on Mainstreaming the Hearing-impaired, the Mentally Retarded and the Visually Handicapped in the Regular Classroom.* Rochester, NY: National Technical Institute for the Deaf.

114 HEMMINGS, I. (1972) 'A survey of units for hearing-impaired children in schools for normally hearing children.' *Teacher of the Deaf,* **70,** 445–66.

115 HEWISON, J. (1980) Address to a conference on teacher-parent collaboration in children's early reading. University of London Institute of Education, 26 April 1980.

116 HEWITT, A. (1977) 'Integration of adult deaf students into colleges of further education.' Lecture at University of London Institute of Education, 15 September 1977.

117 HOLCOMB, R. (1970) 'The total approach.' *Proceedings* of the International Congress on the Education of the Deaf, Stockholm.

118 HOLMBERG, B. (1977) *Distance Education: A Survey and Bibliography.* London: Kogan Page.

119 HUNTINGDON, A. (1981) *Hearing Aids Currently Available.* Manchester: Department of Audiology, University of Manchester.

120 JAMES, J. (1976) *From Where He Stands: A Case Study.* Wellington, N.Z.: New Zealand Department of Education.

121 JAMES, J. (1978) *I Didn't Really Expect to Know.* Wellington, N.Z.: New Zealand Department of Education.

122 JAMES, P. and JAMES, C. (1980) 'The benefits of art for mainstreamed hearing-impaired children.' *Volta Review,* **82,** 103–8.

123 JAMIESON, M., PARLETT, M. and POCKLINGTON, K. (1977) *Towards Integration: A Study of Blind and Partially Sighted Children in Ordinary Schools.* Windsor, Berks.: National Foundation for Educational Research.

124 JOHNSON, E.M. (1963) *A Report on a Survey of Deaf Children Transferred from Special Schools or Units to Ordinary Schools.* London: HMSO.

125 JOHNSON, J.C. (1963) *Educating Hearing-impaired Children in Ordinary Schools.* Manchester: University of Manchester Press.

126 JOHNSON, R.B. and JOHNSON, S.R. (1975) *Towards Individualizing Learning: A Developer's Guide to Self-instruction.* Reading, Mass.: Addison-Wesley.

127 JORDAN, T.E. (1961) 'Historical notes on early study of the deaf.' *Journal of Speech and Hearing Research,* **26,** 118–21.

128 JUSTMAN, J. and MOSKOWITZ, S. (1956) *The Integration of Deaf Children in a Hearing Class.* New York: Board of Education, City of New York (publication no. 36).

129 KAMP, E. (ed.) (1972) 'Integration of hearing handicapped in the community.' In *Proceedings* of the Fourth Danavox Symposium, Elsinore, Denmark. *Scandinavian Audiology,* Supplementum 4.

130 KARCHMER, M.A. and TRYBUS, R.J. (1977) 'Who are the deaf children in mainstream programs?' Research bulletin, series R, no. 4, Office of Demographic Studies, Gallaudet College, Washington, D.C.

131 KARPF, A. (1979) 'Schools that need to be special.' *The Guardian* (London), 4 January 1979.

132 KATZ, L., MATHIS, S.L. and MERRILL, E.C. (1974) *The Deaf Child in the Public Schools: A Handbook for Parents.* Danville, Ill.: Interstate.

133 KELLER, HELEN (1902) *The Story of My Life.* New York: Grosset and Dunlap.

134 KELLY, A.V. (1975) *Case Studies in Mixed Ability Teaching.* London: Harper & Row.

135 KIRK, S.A. (1964) 'Research in education.' In H.A. Stevens and R. Heber (eds) *Mental Retardation: A Review of Research*. Chicago: University of Chicago Press, 57–99.

136 LABON, D. and ACKLAW, J. (1972) Adjustment groups in primary schools. *Therapeutic Education*, Autumn, 32–40.

137 LANE, H. (1977) *The Wild Boy of Aveyron*. London: Allen and Unwin.

138 LANE, H.S. (1976) The profoundly deaf: has oral education succeeded? *Volta Review*, **78**, 329–40.

139 LAWTON, D. (1980) *The Politics of the School Curriculum*. London: Routledge and Kegan Paul.

140 LENNEBERG, E.H. (1967) *Biological Foundations of Language*. London: John Wiley.

141 LING, D. (1976) *Speech and the Hearing-impaired Child: Theory and Practice*. Washington, D.C.: Alexander G. Bell Association for the Deaf.

142 LORING, J. and BURN, G. (eds) (1975) *Integration of Handicapped Children in Society*. London: Routledge and Kegan Paul/Spastics Society.

143 LOVE, H.D. (1972) *Educating Exceptional Children in Regular Classrooms*. Springfield, Ill.: Charles C. Thomas.

144 LÖWE, A. (1972) 'Difficulties facing the integration of hearing-impaired children into regular educational programmes in the Federal Republic of Germany.' In *Proceedings* of the Fourth Danavox Symposium, Elsinore, Denmark. *Scandinavian Audiology*, Supplementum 4.

145 LOWENFELD, B. (1974) *The Visually Handicapped Child in School*. London: Constable.

146 LUNDSTROEM, K. (1978) 'L'integration de l'enfant handicapé en Suède.' *Le Courrier de Suresnes*, **24**, 23–7.

147 LUNZER, E.A. (1966) *The Manchester Scales of Social Adaptation*. Windsor, Berks.: National Foundation for Educational Research.

148 LYNAS, W. (1980) 'The hearing-impaired child in the ordinary school.' *Journal of the British Association of Teachers of the Deaf*, **4**, 2, 49–57.

149 MARSTERS, J.C. Discussions with the author, 1964–79.

150 MARSTERS, J.C. (1979) 'Tuning in to deaf children.' *Dental Management*, July 1979, 40–4.

151 MARTIN, E.W. (1974) 'Some thoughts on mainstreaming.' *Exceptional Children*, **41**, 150–3.

152 MARTIN, J.A.M. and MOORE, W.H. (eds) (1979) 'Childhood deafness in the European Community.' Commission of the European Communities, Medicine Contract No. 359-77-9 ECI UK.

153 MARTIN, NANCY *et al.* (1976) *Writing and Learning Across the Curriculum 11–16* (The Schools Council and University of London Institute of Education Joint Project). London: Ward Lock Educational.

154 MARY, R. (1980) 'Integration of hearing-impaired children in ordinary schools.' *Speak Out* (Madras, India), **3**, 18–20.

155 MACMILLAN, D.L. (1971) 'Special education for the mentally retarded: servant or savant?' *Focus on Exceptional Children*, **2**, 9, 1–11.

156 MCVEAGH, H.E. (1978) *Basic Schooling and Teacher Support in Sparsely Populated Areas: A Case Study of the New Zealand Correspondence School* (OECD/CERI Project). Wellington, N.Z.: Correspondence School Department of Education.

157 MEYEN, E.L. *et al.* (eds) (1972) *Strategies for Teaching Exceptional Children*. Denver, Colo.: Love Publishing Co.

158 Ministry of Education (1963) *A Report on a Survey of Deaf Children Who Have Transferred from Special Schools or Universities to Ordinary Schools.* London: HMSO.

159 MITTLER, P.(ed.) (1977) *Research to Practice in Mental Retardation* (vol. 1). Baltimore, Md.: University Park Press.

160 National Development Group for the Mentally Handicapped (1980) *Helping Mentally Handicapped School Leavers.* London: National Development Group for the Mentally Handicapped.

161 National Education Association Panel (1978) *Education for All Handicapped Children: Consensus, Conflict and Challenge.* Washington, D.C.: National Education Association.

162 National Union of Teachers (1977) *Special Education in Ordinary Schools.* London: National Union of Teachers.

163 NIX, G.W. (ed.) (1976) *Mainstream Education for Hearing-impaired Children and Youth.* New York: Grune and Stratton.

164 NORTHCOTT, W.H. (ed.) (1973) *The Hearing-impaired Child in a Regular Classroom.* Washington, D.C.: Alexander G. Bell Association for the Deaf.

165 NORTHCOTT, W.H. (1979) 'On behalf of parents in the Individualized Education Program (IEP).' *Volta Review*, reprint no. 80-B.

166 NYQUIST, E. (1974) *Mainstreaming: Ideas and Actuality.* Albany, N.Y.: State Education Department.

167 O'CONNOR, C.D. and CONNOR, L.E. (1961) 'Deaf children in regular classrooms.' *Exceptional Children*, **27,** 483-6.

168 OSWIN, M. (1978) *Children Living in Long-stay Hospitals.* London: Heinemann Medical Books.

169 OWRID, H.L. (1960) 'Measuring spoken language in deaf children.' *Teacher of the Deaf*, **58,** 24-34, 124-8.

170 OWRID, H.L. and HAMILTON, P. (1972) 'Comparison of hearing impairment and socio-cultural disadvantage in relation to verbal retardation.' *British Journal of Audiology*, **8,** 27-32.

171 PARFIT, J. (1975) *The Integration of Handicapped Children in Greater London: Report of a Survey for the Institute of Research into Mental and Multiple Handicap.* London: National Bureau for Studies in Child Care.

172 PAYNE, R. and MURRAY, C. (1974) 'Principals' attitudes towards integration of the handicapped.' *Exceptional Children*, **41,** 123-5.

173 PEARSON, E.E. (1977) Personal communication between County Organiser of Audiology, County Hall, Norwich, and author, April 1977.

174 PEARSON, E.E. (1979) 'Happy the tail that has wagged "Dogsbodies".' *Talk*, **92,** 26-7.

175 PIAZZA, R. and NEWMAN, I. (1978) *Readings in Individualized Educational Programs.* Guilford, Conn.: Special Learning Corp.

176 PINEL, P. (1911) Report to the Societé des observateurs de l'homme concerning the child known by the name of 'Sauvage de l'Aveyron'. *Journal of the Society of Anthropology.*

177 PITTENGER, P. (1964) Discussion between Professor Pittenger and the author, San Francisco, April 1964.

178 PLOWDEN, B. (Chair) (1967) *Children and Their Primary Schools: A Report of the Central Advisory Council for Education* (vol. 1). London: HMSO.

179 PORTER, G. (1975) 'The missing vital dimension in successful integration.' *Volta Review*, **77,** 416-22.

180 POULSON, A. (1979) 'An integrated teaching programme for the reading retarded.' *School Psychology*, **1**, 2, 9.

181 PUMFREY, P.D. and SAMPSON, O.C. (1970) 'A study of remedial education in the secondary stage of schooling.' *Remedial Education*, **5**, 102–11.

182 RATTNER, S.L. (1973) 'The way it looks to me: views of an integrated student.' In W.H. Northcott (ed.), *The Hearing-Impaired Child in a Regular Classroom*. Washington, D.C.: Alexander G. Bell Association for the deaf.

183 RAWLINGS, B.W., TRYBUS, R.J. and BISER, J. (1978) *A Guide to College/Career Programs for Deaf Students*. Washington, D.C.: Office of Demographic Studies, Gallaudet College.

184 *Readings from Scientific American: Psychology in Progress* (1975). San Francisco, Calif.: W.H. Freeman.

185 REICH, C., HAMBLETON, D. and KLEIN, B. (1975) *The Integration of Hearing-impaired Children into Regular Classrooms. Research report.* Ontario: Ministry of Education.

186 *Report* (unpublished) to the Ewing Foundation by D.M.C. Dale, London, July 1971.

187 *Report* to the Secretary of Health, Education and Welfare by the Advisory Committee on Education of the Deaf. Washington, D.C., 1965.

188 RIFFER, R. (1970) *1. Student Social Development at NTID. 2. Determinants of the Sociometric Patterns Among Deaf and Hearing Students at NTID.* Rochester, NY: National Technical Institute for the Deaf, Rochester Institute of Technology.

189 RODDA, M. *et al.* (1974) 'Some aspects of the development of young hearing-impaired children.' *American Association of the Deaf*, 121, 391–405.

190 ROSS, M. (1972) *Principles of Aural Rehabilitation*. Indianapolis, Ind.: Bobbs-Merrill.

191 ROSS, M. and GIOLAS, T.G. (eds) (1978) *Auditory Management of Hearing-impaired Children*. Baltimore, Md.: University Park Press.

192 RUSSELL, P. (1978) 'Warnock and after: a parent's view.' *Special Education*, **5**, 7.

193 Russell Report (1973) *Adult Education: A Plan for Development* (report of Committee of Inquiry appointed by the Secretary of State for Education and Science). London: HMSO.

194 RUTTER, M. *et al.* (1979) *Secondary Schools and Their Effects on Children*. London: Open Books.

195 RUTTER, M., TIZARD, J. and WHITMORE, K. (eds) (1970) *Education, Health and Behaviour*. London: Longman.

196 RYOR, J. (1976) 'Mainstreaming' (editorial). *Today's Education*, **65**, 2–5.

197 SALINES, M. (1978) 'Enquête sur les expériences d'integration d'enfants handicapés dans le milieu scolaire normal.' *Le Courrier de Suresnes*, **24**, 52–65.

198 SAMPSON, O.C. (1971) 'Children in a world apart.' *Special Education: Forward Trends*, **60**, June 1971, 6–9.

199 SCHONELL, F.J. (1942) *Backwardness in the Basic Subjects*. Edinburgh: Oliver and Boyd.

200 SCHONELL, F.J. (1955) *Diagnostic and Attainment Testing*. Edinburgh: Oliver and Boyd.

201 SHIELDS, R.W. (1971) *A Cure of Delinquents: The Treatment of Maladjustment*. London: Heinemann.

202 Snowdon Working Party Report (1981) *Integrating the Disabled*. Horsham, West Sussex: National Fund for Research into Crippling Diseases.

203 SPENCER, L.M. (1971) 'The construction of a speech intelligibility test for deaf and partially hearing children.' Unpublished PhD thesis, University of London Institute of Education.
204 SPERRY, L. (ed.) (1972) *Learning Performance and Individual Differences.* Glenview, Ill. and London: Scott, Foresman.
205 STANTON, E.R. Personal communications with the author, May 1976 and January 1980.
206 *Statistics of Education*, vol. I (1974). London: HMSO.
207 STENHOUSE, L. (1975) *An Introduction to Curriculum Research and Development.* London: Heinemann.
208 STEPHEN, R. (1972) 'Living with hearing people.' *Talk*, **63**, 18–21.
209 STONIER, T. (1983) *Wealth of Information: A profile of the post industrial society.* London: Methuen.
210 STOTT, D.H. and MARSTON, N.C. (1971) *Bristol Social Adjustment Guides.* London: Hodder & Stoughton.
211 STRENG, A. (1964) 'The applicability of individualized programmed instruction in the education of deaf children.' *Exceptional Children*, **30**, 365–71.
212 STUCKLESS, E.R. (ed.) (1973) *Principles Basic to the Establishment and Operation of Post-Secondary Education for Deaf Students.* Washington, D.C.: Conference of Executives of American Schools for the Deaf.
213 STUCKLESS, E.R. (1970) 'Research on the social adjustment of NTID students.' *NTID Focus.*
214 STUCKLESS, E.R. and DELGADO, G.L. (1973) *A Guide to College Career Programs for Deaf Students.* Washington, D.C.: NTID and Gallaudet College.
215 SURAN, B.G. and RIZZO, J.V. (1979) *Special Education: An Integrative Approach.* Glenview, Ill., and London: Scott, Foresman.
216 SUTTON, J. (1980) 'Counselling the post-16 hearing-impaired.' *Teacher of the Deaf*, **4**, 89–92.
217 THOMAS, D. (1975) *The Social Psychology of Childhood Disability.* London: Methuen.
218 TIZARD, B. (1975) *Pre-School Education.* Windsor, Berks.: National Foundation for Educational Research.
219 TIZARD, B. and JOSEPH, A. (1970) Cognition development of young children in residential care. *Journal of Child Psychology and Psychiatry*, **2**, 177–86.
220 TIZARD, J. (1967) Foreword. In D.M.C. Dale, *Deaf Children at Home and at School.* London: University of London Press Ltd.
221 TIZARD, J. (1977) Foreword. In C. Cope and E.M. Anderson, *Special Units in Ordinary Schools: An Exploratory Study of Special Provision for Disabled Children* (Studies in Education 6). Windsor, Berks.: National Foundation for Educational Research.
222 TIZARD, J. (1973) 'Maladjusted children and the child guidance service.' In W.D. Wall (ed.), 'The "problem" child – and the psychological services', *London Educational Review*, **2**, 82.
223 TIZARD, J. (1978) Research in special education. *Special Education*, **5**, 3, 23–6.
224 TIZARD, J. and TIZARD, B. (1971) 'The social development of two-year-old children in residential nurseries.' In H.R. Schaffer (ed.), *Origins of Human Social Relations.* London: Academic Press.
225 TOWNSEND, P. (1960) 'The institution and the individual.' *The Listener*, **63**, 1087–9.
226 TREVELYAN, G.M. (1942) *The Illustrated English Social History* (vol. 4). London: Longman.

227 VANDENBERG, M. (1971) 'Children with hearing aids in classes for the normally hearing.' Unpublished report to the Department of Social Administration and Sociology, Victoria University of Wellington, New Zealand.

228 VAN UDEN, A.M.J. (1977) *A World of Language for Deaf Children*. Amsterdam and Lisse: Swets and Zeitlinger.

229 VERNON, P.E. (1967) *The Standardisation of a Graded Word Reading Test*. London: University of London Press Ltd; Scottish Council for Research in Education Publication 12.

230 VISLIE, L. (1980) 'Integration of handicapped children in Italy.' In *Integration of the Handicapped Adolescent*. Paris: CERI.

231 WALL, W.D. (1978) 'The "problem" child.' *Special Education* 5, *London Educational Review*, **2,** 82.

232 WARNOCK, M. (Chair) (1978) *Children with Special Needs*. London: HMSO.

233 WESTBURY, I. and BELLACK, A.A. (1971) *Research into Classroom Processes*. New York: Teachers' College Press.

234 World Health Forum (1981) Health for all by the year 2000. **2.**

235 WRIGHTSTONE, J.W., ARONOW, M.S. and MOSKOWITZ, S. (1963) 'Developing reading test norms for deaf children.' *American Association of the Deaf*, **108,** 311–16.

236 YATER, V.V. (1977) *Mainstreaming of Children with a Hearing Loss: Practical Guidelines and Implications*. Springfield, Ill.: Charles C. Thomas.

237 YOUNG, M., PERRATON, H. JENKINS, J. and DODDS, T. (1980) *Distance Teaching for the Third World*. London: Routledge and Kegan Paul.

238 CORNETT, O.R. (1976) 'Developments in cued speech.' *Proceedings* of the International Congress on Education of the Deaf, Tokyo, 1975. Tokyo, Japan: NWFDC.

Index of Subjects

Main entries in *italics*.

Index of Authors